HOLISTIC
ENDURANCE
TRAINING

Rockridge Press publishes its books in a variety of electronic and print formats. Some content that appears in print may not be available in electronic books, and vice versa.

TRADEMARKS: Rockridge Press and the Rockridge Press logo are trademarks or registered trademarks of Callisto Media Inc. and/or its affiliates, in the United States and other countries, and may not be used without written permission. All other trademarks are the property of their respective owners. Rockridge Press is not associated with any product or vendor mentioned in this book.

Interior & Cover Designer: John Calmeyer
Art Producer: Sue Bischofberger
Editor: Rochelle Torke
Production Editor: Rachel Taenzler

Photography: © OSTILL/ iStock, cover and p. 74; © HuxleyMedia/shutterstock, cover; © Simon Matzinger/ Unsplash, p. i; © Rob and Julia Campbell/Stocksy, pp. ii-iii; © JP Danko/Stocksy, p. vi; © Clem Onojeghuo/Unsplash, p. x; © Brigantine Designs/ Creative Market, pp. 18 and 90; © Giorgio Trovato/Unsplash, p. 36; © PeopleImages/iStock, p. 60; © BraunS/Getty, p. 104; © torwai/iStock, p. 118; © 2019 Helene Dujardin pp. 122-3, 124, 132, 140-1, 142, 154, 158-9, and 164-5.

Author photo by Abby Peek

ISBN: Print 978-1-64611-233-3
eBook 978-1-64611-234-0

R0

HOLISTIC ENDURANCE TRAINING

The Integrated Approach to Thriving as an Athlete

KIM PEEK

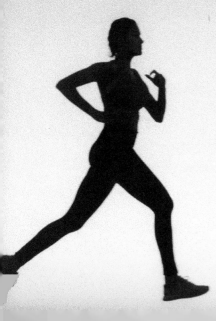

R

ROCKRIDGE PRESS

★ Dad ★

Thank you for teaching me to chase my dreams so I could raise three smart, strong, creative women who pursue theirs.

★ Chris ★

You're still the wind beneath my wings. We've built a pretty amazing team, and I appreciate your never-ending support.

★ Abby, Sarah, and Katie ★

May you forever have the courage to take risks as you share your love, light, and talents with the world. You will always succeed when you follow your heart, do what is right, and treat everyone you encounter with kindness. I'm incredibly proud of each of you, and I know you will go the distance!

CONTENTS

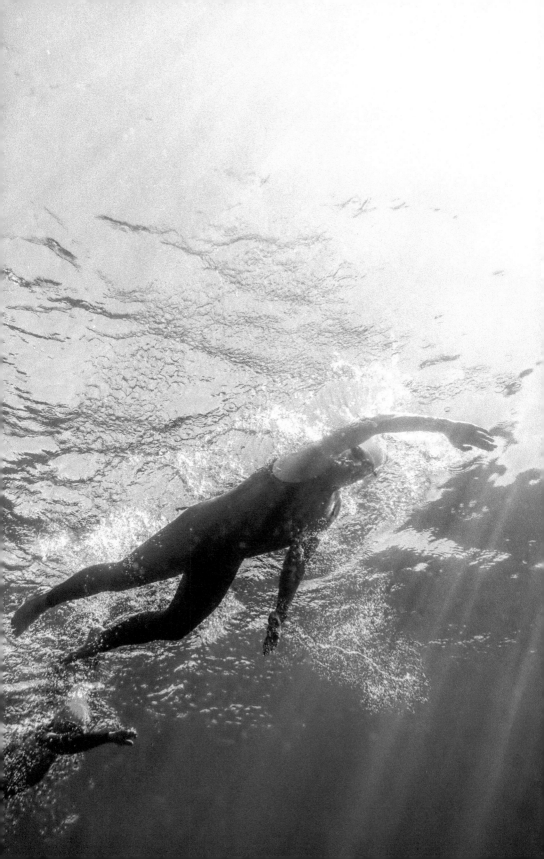

INTRODUCTION

Eleven years ago, as an exhausted mother of three little girls, I began working with a personal trainer named Lucy, who noticed that her clients were lacking in cardiovascular fitness. As part of our small-group training, we ran laps around the gym's track between sets. At the time, I detested running. Every step hurt, my legs felt heavy, and it wasn't even the slightest bit rewarding to me. The track at the gym was one-tenth of a mile, and I could hardly run a full lap. I hated running so much, I threatened to quit working with my trainer if running continued to be part of our biweekly sessions.

I wanted to quit, but my girlfriends had other plans. It's funny how friends step in and give us exactly what we need at just the right time. The sisterhood at my gym was strong, and we had 12 to 16 women who moved in and out of small groups, giving everyone support in the weight room and through life's challenges. Many of these women had run 5Ks and half marathons, so they were up for our trainer's cardio challenge. On the days we didn't work with Lucy, we took group fitness classes together or worked out on our own. My friends often ran on the treadmill, and since I still disliked running, I used the elliptical next to them.

One day, I looked around at the women I spent my time with and noticed how they all looked amazing while I was still carrying the 50 pounds I had gained from giving birth to my girls. I spent significant time at the gym, but I didn't look fit. The one thing my friends were doing that I was not was running. They were doing intense cardio while I was just strolling along. My trainer was right—my cardiovascular fitness was lacking.

In that moment, on the treadmill surrounded by the women I referred to as my "hot mama friends," I decided I would become a runner, too. From that day on, every day they ran, I ran, too. And when I wanted to give up, they pushed me to keep going just a little longer. Whether it was one minute more, or an additional tenth of a mile, my friends encouraged me to keep at it.

This was in January of 2009. I didn't become a runner overnight, but I worked at it consistently. When March rolled around, my friend Amy asked if I'd like to do a 5K with her in April. I agreed, not yet convinced I could finish. By this point, I was losing a lot of weight but still didn't consider myself a runner, so I hadn't yet invested in the array of running gear for every type of weather. Race day was a little chilly, so I grabbed a pair of sweatpants from my closet and met Amy at the race, not realizing that the 40 pounds I'd lost so far meant my pants would be more than a little loose. I spent much of the race holding my pants with one hand because the constant movement made them fall from my hips. Near the end of the race, I wanted to quit, but Amy insisted that we could make it to the finish without stopping to walk. When I crossed the finish line, I was ecstatic—and I was hooked.

Suddenly, I loved running and couldn't get enough. I went overboard, haphazardly increasing my mileage from week to week and racing as often as I could. There might have been people around me at the time who tried to warn me that there was nothing smart about how I trained, but if there were, I wasn't listening to them. I read articles in publications that didn't consistently share quality advice. I tried to emulate the training of more experienced friends. And I found myself competing against them to rack up the most weekly miles. All these practices left me sleep-deprived, overtrained, and with muscle imbalances that led to injury. With amazing quads and a frame that was now 50 pounds lighter, I might have looked like the picture of health, but I was not.

Frustrated by my injured status, I began searching for answers. At the time, there wasn't as much information available in books or online. A friend mentioned that this guy from Newton Running was traveling the country with a gym bag full of shoes. In each city, Danny Abshire, one of Newton's cofounders, partnered with a running store to offer running clinics. Each participant wore a pair of Newtons and learned about running form. When Danny came to Kansas City, Missouri, I went with some friends to see what he could teach us. I learned more about running form in an hour with Danny than I had learned from any source until that point. He mentioned that his company offered a coaching certification, and a group of us got on the mailing list to be notified when registration opened.

I went to Boulder, Colorado, to get my first coaching certification from Newton, which was combined with a certification from the Lydiard Foundation, led by four-time Olympic marathoner Lorraine Moller. I participated in the program because I was seeking answers for myself. My mind was blown, and I couldn't understand why no one was teaching this stuff to recreational runners. I came home determined to seek out additional resources and coaching certifications. I knew I needed to share this life-changing information and help more athletes break out of the injury cycle.

From there, I continued my education, adding certifications, immersing myself in research, and talking to leaders in the field. What I've learned through my studies, and my experiences as a coach and endurance athlete myself, is that we need to slow down and enjoy the scenery. Most of us would benefit from finding more balance with our training, paying attention to the little things, choosing foods that nourish, and treating ourselves with more compassion. I call this kinder, more gentle approach to training responsive endurance training (RET). It's about listening to your body and giving it what it needs.

Your body is trying to get your attention. I've written this book to help you hear what your body is saying. Join me in taking a healthy, powerful, individualized approach to your athletic life. Not every idea I share in this book will work for you—that's the point of the responsive endurance training approach. As you try different strategies, you'll land upon the approach that works best for you. And once you do, it will propel you to the next finish line faster and help you go the distance for a lifetime of healthy athleticism.

CHAPTER 1

A HUMAN APPROACH TO HUMAN BODY TRAINING

ARE YOU READY to learn the most powerful way to perform your best, enjoy the journey, and pursue your athletic passions for life?

In this chapter, I'll introduce you to responsive endurance training, a powerful way to train for and reach your full athletic potential. If you're like me, you love the athletic lifestyle and appreciate the multitude of ways endurance activities enhance your life. Whether you're training so you can take off with a group of friends for a weekend of food, fun, and racing, or you aspire to qualify for an elite race like the Boston or New York City marathon, I bet your life changed the moment you committed to training for an endurance event.

For many endurance junkies, the thrill goes beyond racing: It's the community, the common goals, and that rush you get after achieving something you previously thought was impossible. And once you get a taste of the endurance life, you'll never want the ride to end.

Whether you've been on this journey for decades or you're just getting started, you'll learn techniques that will enhance your performance today—and protect your body so you're capable of participating in endurance sports for many years to come.

What Is Responsive Endurance Training?

Responsive endurance training (RET) means taking an intuitive, holistic, self-study approach to your training, racing, and life. It's important to know yourself and your body. You've probably been told to listen to your body since the first day you started your athletic journey, but have you ever stopped to think about what that really means? How do you know when to trust the messages your body sends you, and how do you even know what your body is trying to say?

Responsive endurance training respects that each body is different. So rather than attempting to apply one-size-fits-all formulas or rules for building athleticism, this method is about taking a scientific approach by testing concepts and studying the results. I'll encourage you to study your training, nutrition, rest, stress, and even social interactions so you can begin to find connections between your habits, the environment you create, and the results you achieve with your training. In the back of this book, you'll find a sample training journal (see page 119), along with prompts and instructions for creating your own journal to track your activities and your body's response to those activities.

Throughout this book, I'll show you how athletic performance is a reflection of total mind-and-body vitality. The way your body performs is not limited to traditional training activities alone. It's more than the time you spend swimming, biking, running, rowing, or climbing. You won't achieve your goals without spending significant time mastering your sport; however, the *little things* like how you respond to stress, the way you talk to yourself when training gets tough, and the influences you allow into your life are significant. Responsive endurance training is a total mind-and-body approach to training.

I will challenge you to move beyond thinking of training as only an athletic pursuit. If you want to surpass your previous limits, it's time to take a holistic approach. You'll see results throughout this training cycle—and most importantly, you'll experience longevity in the sport. While everyone experiences setbacks and injuries—it's part of learning how to listen to the messages your body sends you—the habits you'll develop as you apply the lessons in this book will make you a stronger, more resilient athlete.

It may seem like I'm asking a lot of you. After all, you're probably an endurance athlete because you love endorphins and truly enjoy pushing your limits as you train and race. You might feel overwhelmed when I propose rounding out your training program with some additional rest and recovery tools instead of adding another physical activity. I understand this can be a concern when you're already crunched for time and you're trying to figure out how to squeeze in that long run between your kid's soccer game and the company picnic.

So, let's make a deal: By the time you are done with this book, I want you to have a rainbow of colored notes in the margins. As you read, use one color to highlight the changes you can painlessly make now, and then choose other colors to highlight the behaviors you can work into your life 30, 60, or 90 days from now.

At the beginning of the year, when it's time for New Year's resolutions, people make plans to completely overhaul their lives. Maybe you've found yourself in this position once or twice, and if so, you know what happens next.

It's almost impossible to make grand, sweeping changes and expect them to stick long-term. Despite our best intentions, they're usually not sustainable. While we used to think change was just a matter of willpower, most experts now agree that willpower has limited influence. That means environment and habit are critical to long-term success.

If you are committed to going the distance, you'll learn to develop patience for the long game. You might think you are one of the special people who can do it all, who can immediately overhaul how you live and train. If that's you, do me a favor. Schedule a time to come back to this paragraph in a month. Literally, open your phone and schedule an appointment.

I'm serious. I'm asking a lot of you and, as a coach, I've seen people give up repeatedly. The most sustainable way to develop a training routine that you will maintain is to adopt one new behavior at a time. It might seem tedious, but I assure you that it's quicker than stopping and starting dozens of times. If you stumble, please come back to the book and start again. Add one change at a time—gradually—until you have the balance in your life to do all the things you want to do for your training.

If you've ever met me in person, you might say that optimism is my middle name. So why did I just go down a negative path, telling you exactly how you'll fail? I want to get your attention because I see this happen all the time. Lack of patience is an underlying problem for nearly every athlete I've ever watched give up on themselves.

Here's what I mean. When someone embarks on a new training plan, they are filled with excitement about the training process at the beginning. They follow the plan to the letter for the first two to three weeks, and then reality sets in. Eventually, it gets hard to balance life and training. They skip a workout because of a sick kid or an unscheduled work meeting. And from there, they lose control of their schedule, and the plan begins to unravel. As the guilt piles up, their training becomes sporadic. They miss a workout, so they try to make up for it by doubling and tripling miles on the weekend. This behavior leads to burnout and injury—and does nothing to maximize performance.

Instead, if we learn to be kind to ourselves, if we layer new habits one by one, the way we've successfully added other routines into our lives, we will eventually incorporate each behavior that is necessary to take athletic performance to the next level.

As you move through the book, I'll ask you to heighten your sensitivity to your body, mind, and emotions. You'll plan for success by developing new habits one at a time. You'll teach yourself to have compassion and accept what you can do today, without the added weight of guilt. You'll listen to the feedback you get from your body, and you'll learn to adapt your plan accordingly.

Self-Study Mind-Set

Responsive endurance training is a commitment to observe and listen to your body. Feedback from your nervous system should not be ignored. If you want to achieve your personal best and derive joy from your athletic pursuits, the whole body must be brought on board effectively. If you want to get faster so you can crush your neighbor in the local 5K, you'll be better served by saving the competition for race day—and adopting a daily practice of self-study. It is important to keep your motivation within your own experience. You are now your own experiment of one.

While we know the major practices that will help us excel, there is no magic formula. What helps your neighbor row his best might not work for you. When I first started running, I followed the advice of my more experienced friends. It worked for a while, but as I gained endurance, I found myself wanting to keep up with my Boston Marathon–qualified friends. I pushed my mileage. I cut out rest days. I eliminated strength training. If my friends ran 50 miles in a week, I ran 51. If they cranked a 7:30 pace, I tried for 7:29. I emulated their training and thought that the secret to success was pushing harder.

As you might have guessed, that mentality led to injury. Instead of crossing the finish line with them, I was cheering on the sidelines because my training was cut short. I cannot stress enough the importance of tailoring your training to your body's response. The mantra "no pain, no gain" has become synonymous with excellence. We've been taught that to achieve great things, we must push until it hurts, that pain is a badge of honor. This "no pain, no gain, push until it hurts, and push some more" stance is not part of the responsive endurance training approach.

While endurance sports always entail testing your body's limits, reaching maximum fitness capacity doesn't call for employing that mentality at all times. Part of learning RET is learning how to incorporate the right rest at the right time and to evaluate how your mind and body feel as a result.

In each chapter, you'll find questions that encourage you to check in with yourself. Use these questions, along with your training journal, to reflect on how your training is going. You'll track your rest, recovery, nutrition, mind-set, stress, sport-specific training, mobility routines, strength development, and more.

As you develop a habit of noting the details of your day, you'll see patterns emerge. Endurance athletes around the world thrive on a variety of diets and lifestyles, and it's important to remember that each body is unique. Your body might need more recovery time, less speed work, or a longer training cycle than your cousin's body does. And you'll definitely find that your stomach tolerates prerace meals and training fuels differently than the way your running partner's stomach experiences the exact same nutrition strategies.

This isn't like a high school science test where I can give you a study guide and tell you exactly which facts to regurgitate on an essay. Improving your endurance is an individual experience, and the ultimate test is race day. I don't want you to merely pass this test. I want you to sail through! You'll use what you've discovered about your body's response to everything we're incorporating—training, fuel, recovery, and mind-set strategies—along with what you've learned about how the activities of daily living affect your performance.

This information will inform your training, so you can begin to experiment. Maybe you notice that you're sluggish during your

Tuesday morning training sessions. As you go through your journal, perhaps you see a pattern emerge:

> Your Monday tends to be hectic, and you feel like you're constantly behind. You need more energy, so you reach for another cup of coffee (*with an extra shot of espresso*) at 2:00 p.m. After work, you keep charging hard. There's dinner to make, errands to run, homework to help with, and a load of towels that must be washed so the kids aren't air-drying their bodies by streaking through the house in the morning. At the end of the day, you lie in your bed, staring at the ceiling. You can't sleep, and your alarm is set to go off at 5:00 a.m. so you can meet your training partners for a speed session at the track.

It's no wonder you're sluggish! You're not getting enough rest.

Could it be the 2:00 p.m. coffee that's keeping you awake? Test that theory.

Could it be your never-ending to-do list? See what you can do to relieve some of the pressure.

Could you benefit from a calming evening routine that enhances sleep? Give it a try!

Again, there is no magic formula. The secret is really to learn strong observation skills as you apply ideas from this book. Some of the things you'll track will be subjective, like your mood, your energy, and how you feel. And others will be measurable, such as your heart rate, your hours of sleep, and the pace, distance, and duration of your workout.

Like any good scientist, you'll learn to identify patterns, and you'll form hypotheses. You'll make educated guesses based on how your body responds as you alter variables related to your life and training. This is a work in progress. Your body will respond differently as you go through different seasons of life—but once you get the hang of RET, you'll have the necessary tools to tweak your approach and respond to life's peaks and valleys.

WHY WE RACE

THE HUMAN HISTORY OF RACING FOR PLEASURE

Perhaps you've heard the story of Pheidippides, the professional running courier who ran for over two days straight to carry critical messages during the war between Greece and Persia. Finally, he ran from the town of Marathon to Athens in 490 BCE to announce the decisive Greek victory. As he declared, "Rejoice, we conquer," he fell to the ground and took his dying breath. This famous runner is credited with inspiring countless generations of runners and the creation of the marathon itself as a foot race.

While this is a popular tale—and is often retold by non-runners who question the sanity of running marathons—it is likely more myth than fact. Historians in the fifth century BCE did not mention Pheidippides, and it's possible the legend combines multiple stories to create the hero's tale we are so fond of today.

The first Olympic marathon was 24.8 miles, and the distance for subsequent races fluctuated between 24.8 and 26.2 miles before it was standardized in 1924.

At the 1908 games in London, England, the race was 26.2 miles for the first time, and there are varying stories regarding how that distance was settled on. The race began at Windsor Castle and ended in the Olympic stadium. Some sources say that the start was lengthened so the royal children could see this part of the race from the nursery, and the end was extended so the race would finish in front of the royal box inside the stadium. However, that has been disputed by Bob Wilcock, a historian of the Olympics.

Even after the London Olympics, the marathon distance varied. Some believe the dramatic ending of the 1908 games contributed to the mystique surrounding the distance. Sir Arthur Conan Doyle, the author of the Sherlock Holmes books, wrote about the race for the *Daily Mail*, calling the marathon "the breaker of men."

The first person to finish was Dorando Pietri, a pastry chef who collapsed and was helped across the finish line by an official. The "no outside assistance" rule we know today was already in existence, so he was disqualified. American Johnny Hayes was declared the winner.

Inspired by the success of the marathon in the 1896 Olympics, Massachusetts held its first Boston Marathon on April 19, 1897. It is held on the third Monday of April each year and is the oldest annual marathon. The first Boston Marathon was 24.5 miles. This marathon was lengthened to 26.2 miles in 1924 to match the Olympic standard.

For decades, major running welcomed men only. In 1966, Roberta Gibb was the first woman to run the Boston Marathon, unofficially running alongside thousands of registered male participants. A year later, Kathrine Switzer became the first woman to officially register and race, after registering under her initials, K. V. Switzer. Her own coach initially discouraged her from running, telling her the race was too much for a "fragile woman," before conceding that if any woman could do it, Kathrine could. After she donned her racing number and ran the early miles of the race, event coordinators shouted at her and attempted to extract her from the race by force. She and her boyfriend, a fellow runner, fought back and she continued to run, ultimately changing perceptions of what women were capable of.

The Boston Marathon didn't officially open to women until 1972. Although Kathrine Switzer's bold action paved the way for women in sports, it took another 18 years until women were allowed to compete in the Olympic marathon.

Endurance for Life— through the Best and Worst of Times

One of the goals of RET is to help you develop the behaviors you'll need so you can engage in your favorite activities for life. I remember when I first started racing, I would always chat with runners I saw at the start line, asking them questions about how long they had been racing and their goals for the day. Inevitably, someone in the group would share that they'd been racing for 20 years, but because of a knee injury or a lifetime of racing, their goal for the day was to take it all in and enjoy the scenery.

At the time, it struck me as sad. Who would choose to race without a goal of crushing their previous times? As I've gotten older and gained perspective, I see more value in training for life. As situations and circumstances change, it truly fills my life with joy to continue to train for endurance events.

In the summer of 2015, I was diagnosed with breast cancer. At the time of my diagnosis, I was in the best shape of my life and had my eye on qualifying for USA Triathlon Age Group Nationals. Leading up to my bilateral mastectomy, I trained and raced hard—a choice that no doubt provided me with the mental and physical strength I needed for recovery.

As I recovered, I surrounded myself with friends who were willing to go for long walks and talk, providing the exercise and support I craved. A few weeks later, I found out I would need chemotherapy, so I set a goal of completing a 5K for each round of chemo and celebrating the last of my treatments with a half marathon. These goals helped me focus on something bigger than the pain of surgery and chemo. On my good days, I trained. On the bad days, I rested. And I always listened to my body, accepting where I was at the time—and what my body was capable of in any given moment.

What does this story have to do with endurance for life? It shows how you can incorporate RET into your life every day, especially when times are tough. RET is about listening to your body, being kind to yourself, accepting where you are, all while staying focused on a goal.

Because I had a hormone-positive form of cancer, one that feeds off estrogen, I am on a hormone-blocking drug that sucks every last bit of estrogen out of my body. Each person has a different response to therapies, and in my case, this drug has caused severe joint pain, and, early on, hot flashes, brain fog, and memory issues that affected my ability to work.

However, because I am passionate about running and the benefits of exercise for the brain, I have not let these obstacles get in my way. Instead, I applied the principles of RET so that I can continue to enjoy training, racing, and the friendships my sports have brought into my life. In addition to taking a more body-friendly approach to my training, I incorporated mobility and flexibility work, and strength training. I honored the value of rest and recovery. I also acknowledged that mind-set is critical to performance. And, of course, I continued to pay attention to how I fueled my body, focusing on foods that energized my activities and also reduced inflammation.

My story isn't unique. Everyone will encounter something that disrupts their life at some point. And when that time comes, you will have a choice: Will you let the disruption ruin you, or will you rise to the challenge and focus on the things you have control over? You can have a lifetime of athleticism when you learn to observe what is going on with your body and how to adapt to what you notice and pace yourself accordingly.

Can You Have Too Much of a Good Thing?

The health benefits of endurance sports cannot be denied. However, it's important to recognize when you're veering into unhealthy territory. When running crosses into an obsession or an addiction, it has the potential to damage your health. Just as too much running can cause an overuse injury such as shin splints or Achilles tendinitis, some medical professionals believe your heart can also experience adverse effects from extreme levels of high-intensity exercise.

Several studies have shown that excessive endurance training can cause serious cardiovascular issues. I am sharing this research not to scare you but to help you evaluate the risks and benefits so you can make informed decisions about the intensity and duration of your training activities.

One of the most famous studies is from a 2012 paper (and a related TEDx Talk that has over one million views) by cardiologist Dr. James H. O'Keefe and colleagues, which showed that "long-term excessive endurance exercise may induce pathologic structural remodeling of the heart and large arteries. . . . Additionally, long-term excessive sustained exercise may be associated with coronary artery calcification, diastolic dysfunction, and large-artery wall stiffening." The research received a lot of attention and has been a source of controversy, with many people wondering if the physical and mental rewards are worth the risk.

The risk of dying from a heart attack in a race is one in 100,000. "One in 100,000 is a pretty low risk, but I'm not so worried about that," Dr. O'Keefe says in his TEDx Talk. "Running is supposed to add years to your life, and even life to your years. Could it be shortening your life expectancy? I'm not worried about dropping in a race. I'm just trying to do the right thing. I'm a cardiologist. I'm in the business of finding out the ideal diet and lifestyle. I'm coming to the conclusion that running marathons and extreme endurance athletics do not fit into that recipe."

For sure, this is not the type of research an endurance junkie wants to read. Everyone agrees that exercise is beneficial. That is not disputed. Physicians, scientists, and athletes have debated this research for years, and although there is disagreement regarding the statistics, most researchers agree there is a point at which the athlete will experience diminishing returns—and *could* experience adverse cardiovascular effects.

So, how do we define excessive exercise?

According to the original study, "Running distances of about 1 to 20 miles per week, speeds of 6 to 7 miles per hour, and frequencies of 2 to 5 days per week were associated with lower all-cause mortality, whereas higher mileage, faster paces, and more frequent runs were not associated with better survival."

I spoke with Dr. O'Keefe while writing this book, and he provided some additional guidelines that might help recreational runners satisfy their need for endurance while guarding their heart health.

Guidelines from Dr. O'Keefe

* Training for longevity means keeping the majority of your exercise in the light-to-moderate intensity range, also known as the Goldilocks Zone.
* Pace and heart rate vary from person to person, so the talk test is a good guide for judging intensity. If you can't maintain a conversation while exercising, that's a strenuous workout. A heart-pounding, sweat-producing workout is also considered strenuous. If it's less than that, you can consider the workout moderate. A light workout is any workout where you hardly notice an increase in your heart rate.
* There is no upper limit for moderate physical activity, such as gardening, walking, and housework, or for active play, such as golf, racquet sports, billiards, bowling, and dancing.
* Limit strenuous activity to two and a half hours or less a week.

* If you're over 40, limit high-intensity intervals to no more than once a week.
* Diversify your physical activities by mixing high-intensity activities like running with lower-intensity movement such as yoga, Pilates, walking, and hiking.
* Enjoy a day of rest each week.

Dr. O'Keefe also encourages us to play. "Mammals invented physical, interactive play about 80 million years ago, and it is our remedy for stress and anxiety, the best way to socially bond, and it's a great way to hone your physical survival skills in the real world," he says. The idea that exercise should be social, rewarding, and fun is not new. It is well established that we are more consistent when we engage in exercise that we look forward to. If the goal of responsive endurance training is to train in a way that we can maintain for life, we should give these recommendations serious consideration.

We will touch on the importance of social interaction again later in the book, but Dr. O'Keefe made a critical point during our discussion. "The social connection, emotional support, and social network we build around us is the most important thing for long-term health and well-being, mental and physical health," he said. "Physical interactive play is a really unique and powerful way to cultivate friendships." The takeaway: Rather than training alone, find a training partner or group—and make friends. Social interaction is phenomenal for your health, and it's a way to improve consistency in your training.

While it is important to be aware of the risks of excessive endurance training, you should also know that the risks of too little exercise are a far bigger problem. Regular exercise increases life expectancy by up to six years, and a lifelong habit of regular physical activity is one of the most effective approaches for enhancing longevity and health.

We need a combination of cardiovascular exercise and strength training—and the vast majority of adults in the United States do not meet the guidelines established by the Centers for Disease Control and Prevention.

For those of you who still have some doubt about Dr. O'Keefe's guidelines, or who are inclined to train without reducing the duration or intensity of your routine, later in the book I will show you how to apply heart-smart principles, backed by research, that will improve your aerobic capacity and endurance.

I find Dr. O'Keefe's research compelling, but skeptics might prefer to read some of the studies that refute his research on the dangers of excessive endurance training. You can find these studies, as well as additional thoughts and links to the studies cited, in the References section of this book.

Endurance training is clearly a hotly debated topic, and research will continue to change our thinking.

Getting the Most from This Book

It's no secret that endurance athletes can be intense. Running can help manage symptoms of depression, help us sort through problems, and provide us with an important social outlet. When injury or illness gets in the way and disrupts the training cycle, life can be emotionally challenging. In addition to missing out on an activity that helps manage stress, anxiety, and depression, the athlete may feel isolated.

While recovering from a setback, you may feel like your teammates have moved on without you. You feel left out of all the fun and miss out on new bonding activities and inside jokes. When your sport is such a big part of your life, you can feel lost and a little helpless when it is suddenly gone.

I know you want to maximize your performance, and to do that you need to be consistent with your training. Being consistent

BE GOOD ᴛᴏ YOURSELF

It's time for an emotional check-in. This connection between the mind and body is a core concept behind responsive endurance training. The mind is powerful, and the way we think can be one of the biggest predictors of, or limitations to, success.

A study in *Nature Human Behaviour* by Dr. Bradley P. Turnwald and colleagues demonstrated that beliefs about athletic ability shape our reality. The CREB1 gene is a strong predictor of endurance potential, and as part of the study, subjects were told either they had the variant of this gene linked to poor exercise capacity or that their body could tolerate a high level of exercise. Subjects first completed a treadmill test without knowing their genetic risk. Upon learning whether they had the genetic variant (randomly assigned, not their true risk), the subjects completed an additional treadmill test.

Results of the study showed that receiving genetic risk information affected the subjects' physiology. Subjects who believed they had a genetic variant making them less responsive to exercise had cardiorespiratory, endurance, and perceived exertion responses that reflected poor exercise capacity.

In other words, their beliefs directly affected their athletic ability. Because they believed they had the genetic variant, it became a self-fulfilling prophecy. In some cases, the physiological effects were greater than what should be caused by the actual genetic variant.

What does this tell us about how we train and perform on race day? It means we perform to the level of our expectations. Athleticism is a total mind-and-body undertaking, so it is important to check in with yourself regarding any limiting beliefs you may have about your athletic potential, your training, and your abilities. Be selective of the thoughts that you allow into your head, as well as the influences in your life. There is truth to the saying "What we think, we become."

means taking care of your body and giving it what it needs so you aren't sidelined with a serious injury.

Living the endurance lifestyle can be a huge ego boost. You know you are strong. You understand the power of the mind. And you participate in activities that your friends and acquaintances might think are superhuman. As an endurance athlete, you feel like you're on top of the world because you have developed the ability to test your limits and push yourself further than you ever imagined was possible.

It's because of the personality traits that make you successful that I say this: There is a better way.

As you read this book, I want you to think about a kinder way to train. A way of training that respects your current health and fitness level and the stress in your life. A way of training where you are encouraged to take a complete mind-and-body approach. Your key workouts will be the most important activities of the week. You can't excel without sport-specific training, so I'm not suggesting you give that up. However, I do want you to look at factors that we tend to think of as supplemental (e.g., yoga, strength, mobility, rest, mind-set, and nutrition), and consider them *nonnegotiable* parts of your training.

By taking a holistic approach to your training, you'll participate in a healthy mind-and-body growth process that factors your unique physiology and mental state into the equation. Read the chapters of this book in order so you can see how each subsequent concept builds on the one preceding it. As you adopt RET, you'll do away with one-size-fits-all training programs. You'll learn to examine your behaviors and you'll discover how your actions affect your athletic performance as well as how you show up for yourself on a daily basis.

CHAPTER 2

THE
HEART
OF THE
MATTER

IN THIS CHAPTER, we will talk about how to use heart rate training to improve your performance and maximize your potential while being mindful of the possible risks of excessive endurance activity. Because cardiovascular health plays a huge role in overall wellness and life expectancy, it is critical to every aspect of endurance training. You'll learn how to increase your aerobic capacity with key workouts, and you'll come away with training strategies that offer alternatives to the monotony and pain of grinding out brutal sweaty sessions *day after day after day*. I am not advocating that you rely solely on low-intensity training, but I am asking you to keep an open mind and consider the possibility that there is a place in your plan for a variety of paces and exertion levels.

Measuring Exertion

If improved aerobic capacity helps build endurance, it makes sense to have a means of monitoring the intensity of our workouts. There are three primary ways you can measure exertion when you train: heart rate, rate of perceived exertion (RPE), and pace. I believe they each have a place, and at different times, you'll use each of these methods to gain valuable feedback.

In your training journal, you'll want to track one or more of these rates with each workout so you can start to identify patterns. An elevated heart rate could point to overtraining, lack of sleep, fatigue, stress, or dehydration, or it could mean the weather was especially hot or humid on a particular day. A decreased heart rate—if the route, weather conditions, and pace are the same—might mean your body is responding to the training and your heart is getting stronger.

First, let's look at what we mean by heart rate, pace, and RPE. Then, we'll discuss how to measure each.

Heart Rate Training

A heart rate monitor can help you assess your exertion level objectively in order to maximize a training effect. Most athletes inadvertently spend too much time in the gray zone, the area between high and low intensity that provides little training effect. We gravitate to this middle ground because it's just hard enough to make us sweat and feel like we're getting a good workout. However, the problem with spending too much time here is that it may create enough fatigue to inhibit future workouts without actually boosting our aerobic capacity. Instead, pursuing some bursts of higher intensity, heart rate–spiking activity strengthens the cardiovascular system without provoking deep fatigue.

> **PRO** Heart rate training will help you listen to your body so you'll train within an appropriate zone. It can help you gauge the progress you are making when you compare various sessions in

similar conditions (weather, route, distance, plus your own personal factors such as sleep, fatigue, hydration, and stress). And it provides information that will help you stay within an appropriate zone when you are in situations where heart rate is affected. I especially like to measure heart rate, rather than pace, in the hot summer months when you might be tempted to stick with a pace goal since hot weather affects intensity. Rather than feel defeated because you didn't achieve a particular pace in challenging conditions, I want you to know the workout was still effective.

CON Heart rate training is based on max heart rate (MHR) or lactate threshold, and it can be challenging to discover your true numbers without being tested in a lab. Not all heart rate monitors are accurate, and most methods of calculating max heart rate and lactate threshold on your own can be confusing. Because there is a lag between your actual heart rate and what the monitor picks up, the monitor is unreliable when you are exercising for short intervals. Finally, to use this method, you'll need a watch or device that tracks heart rate.

Pace

Your pace—the speed at which you move—can be a good measure of your current fitness level, but it can vary greatly with weather, sleep, hydration, and stress. Pace gives you an idea of the progress you've made and how consistently you're performing. For example, do you start out blazing fast and then slow to a snail's pace near the end of the race? Are you getting consistent mile splits? If speed drops off near the end, it can be a sign that endurance is lacking, or that there is another factor affecting performance.

PRO Pace gives an athlete a way to compare information from session to session. If a runner did a time trial on the same route, with similar weather, two months apart, and cut five minutes from their time, we could assume that their fitness improved. By using pace, we can use a one-mile or 5K time to predict the length of time it would take to complete a longer race. And we can also use

Zone	% of Max Heart Rate	RPE	Talk Test	
1	50–60%	1–3	Can speak in full sentences; a good walking pace	
2	60–70%	4–5	Conversational; could exercise all day at this pace	
3	70–80%	6–7	Speaking a sentence at a time; a tougher workout	
4	80–90%	8–9	One or two words at a time, max; comfortably hard effort	
5	90% +	10	Too hard to talk; very hard effort	

When to Use	Benefit
Warm up, cool down, walking	Physiological adaptations such as increased mito-chondrial density, increased number of strokes, increased number of capillaries, increased blood volume. The body uses mostly fat to create energy.
Long run, ride, or row; recovery run, ride, or row; base building	
Good as a recovery heart rate between intervals; most endurance athletes spend too much time here	This is a gray zone where you will still benefit, but you may find you go too hard on an easy day or too easy on a hard day and don't get the training adaptation your plan was trying to achieve. Carbs and fats are used for energy.
Use this for workouts designed to increase your lactate threshold so you can run, cycle, swim, or row at higher intensities for longer periods of time. Tempo runs, fartleks, and longer intervals are done at this rate.	The body gets better at using carbohydrates for energy. At this rate, you increase lac-tate threshold and improve speed endurance.
Aerobic intervals, short bursts, speed. (The work will take place too quickly for the HR monitor to accurately track.)	Workouts at this intensity are designed to increase your VO_2 max (maximal oxygen uptake).

this information to create a pacing strategy for a longer race so that an athlete starts at a pace they can maintain throughout the event.

C O N To track pace, you'll want a sports watch for the greatest accuracy. While it is possible to use an app on your phone, the GPS can sometimes lag, making the pace measurement unreliable. Some athletes become too dependent on their technology and push their body to its limits, no matter the circumstances.

Rate of Perceived Exertion

The rate of perceived exertion (RPE) is just that. How hard do you perceive you're working? RPE can be used along with the talk test to gauge the intensity of a workout. During an easier workout, you'll be able to speak in complete sentences. Once you cross beyond a moderate pace, you'll be able to get only a few words out at a time. Higher intensity means you can utter a word between gasps, and at the highest intensity, you'll feel more like puking than speaking.

P R O RPE and the talk test do not require technology or gadgets. RPE is all based on how you feel. And, ultimately, running by feel is what is best for your body.

C O N This method is subjective and doesn't provide hard numbers to analyze. Ideally, you would use RPE or the talk test in conjunction with pace or heart rate data so you can get a more detailed picture of how your training is going.

Understanding Heart Rate Zones

Responsive endurance training encourages training in a way that gives you longevity in your sport. By combining heart rate, RPE, and talk test data, you'll learn to understand the signals your body sends regarding your training. If you look online for a heart rate training plan, you'll find a variety of confusing plans—and many don't match the data you get from your watch or tracking device. To keep things simple, cross-check the information you receive from your tracking device with the five-zone system explained in the table on page 22.

A Super Quick Overview about How to Apply This

In the early stages of training, while you are building your base, you will spend the majority of your time in zones 1 and 2. This might feel really odd at first, and you might have difficulty keeping your heart rate in that range. However, with patience, you'll soon see that your speed increases while your heart rate remains in the same zones. You will notice that your fitness is improving, and your heart is not having to work as hard to maintain the same pace.

As you progress through your training plan, you will add intensity in the form of fartlek runs, tempo runs, and speed work. As you move beyond your base phase and are physically prepared for more challenging workouts, you will work in zone 4 or 5 up to 20 percent of the time (or using Dr. O'Keefe's guidelines, no more than two and a half hours a week). While you can certainly train in zone 3, you will find that your time is better spent in the other zones.

Understanding Max Heart Rate

Max heart rate (MHR) is an estimate of the maximum number of beats per minute that your heart is capable of. For the most accurate test, you would go to a lab and perform a treadmill test under the supervision of an exercise physiologist. Most people don't have access to a lab or aren't able to expend the time or money for the test.

The standard MHR formula, 220 minus your age, is likely the formula used by your treadmill and your tracking devices. However, we are all *individuals*, and the problem with using a generic

WHY WE RACE

COMPETITIVE INTEGRITY

In our quest to test the limits of human performance, we may tinker with nutrition, test new shoes, or experiment with caffeine or other fuels. But what happens when athletes adopt a win-at-all-costs mentality?

You've probably heard stories of runners who find ways to cut the course, or hop in a taxi for a leisurely couple of miles, all to place in their age group. Or maybe you've seen stories about people who get a faster friend to wear their bib for the purpose of recording a Boston-qualifying time.

The ways that people cheat can be elaborate, ultimately denying someone of a placement or qualifying slot that has been earned. Whether it's finding ways to cheat on the course or using performance-enhancing drugs, there is no room in sport for cheaters.

In September 2019, a four-year investigation into representatives at the Nike Oregon Project came to a head when two independent three-member panels of the American Arbitration Association determined that head coach Alberto Salazar and a consultant, Dr. Jeffrey Brown, "trafficked testosterone, a banned performance-enhancing substance, administered a prohibited IV infusion, and engaged in tampering to attempt to prevent relevant information about their conduct from being learned by [the US Anti-Doping Agency (USADA)]."

According to a statement in the press release from USADA Chief Executive Officer Travis T. Tygart, "The athletes in these cases found the courage to speak out and ultimately exposed the truth. . . . While acting in connection with the Nike Oregon Project, Mr. Salazar and Dr. Brown demonstrated that winning was more important than the health and well-being of the athletes they were sworn to protect."

Both Salazar and Brown denied any wrongdoing, and Nike stood behind its coach, although they did shut down the Nike Oregon Project, which Salazar led.

Less than two months after this ruling came down, the *New York Times* ran a heart-wrenching opinion piece by Mary Cain, an athlete who trained under Salazar. In the video "I Was the Fastest Girl in America, Until I Joined Nike," Cain says, "I joined Nike because I wanted to be the best female athlete ever. Instead, I was emotionally and physically abused by a system designed by Alberto and endorsed by Nike."

Called a high school track phenom by *Sports Illustrated*, Cain joined the Nike Oregon Project while she was still in high school. Eventually, at 23, she began speaking out about the focus on her weight, public weigh-ins, emotional abuse, and pressure to use banned substances. She says that even when she told Salazar that she'd become depressed and was cutting herself, the program offered no support. Cain left the program in October 2016 but spoke publicly about her experience for the first time in November 2019.

Olympian Kara Goucher, a whistle-blower in the Salazar case, was quick to come to Cain's defense, reminding the athletic community that Cain's case is another example of the abusive culture that must be addressed. Goucher has become a champion for clean sport and has launched a podcast where she and her cohosts, Shanna Burnette and Chris McClung, talk with athletes, brands, and coaches about the issues surrounding clean sport.

While recreational runners rarely have prize money, sponsorships, or a shot at the Olympics on the line, it's important to compete ethically. As we become more aware of issues in the sport, we are better equipped to support fellow athletes and speak out when we see ethics and clean-sport violations.

formula to calculate your training zones is that if the zone isn't customized to you, the effort doesn't match the intended zone. So when you think you're working in zone 3, you could be in zone 2 or 4. That doesn't mean you won't benefit from the work. It just means that a particular workout might not be training in the zone in which you set out to train.

In short: Generic formulas do not take into account individual differences such as genetics, gender, age, and medications—all of which could affect MHR.

How should you determine your MHR? The best way would be to perform a test under medical supervision. However, the next best way is to enlist the help of a friend and conduct your own test. **Remember that if you have not been exercising or are not in peak shape, it is not safe to do an all-out test to determine your max heart rate.**

If you are new to exercising, you would be wise to spend six to eight weeks using the RPE scale and training based on how you feel. Your MHR will vary from sport to sport, which means you will want to calculate your MHR for each sport where you are tracking your heart rate.

Ways of Calculating Your Max Heart Rate

5K RACE TEST Complete a 5K race or make up your own course and complete a time trial. As you enter the last two minutes of the event, race all out to the finish. Note your heart rate at the end. This number should be close to your max heart rate.

HIGHEST NOTED RATE If you've done a lot of exercise with a heart rate monitor, you might be fascinated by the highest numbers you observe on your tracking device as you perform speed work. While taking my favorite treadmill class, I have surpassed my highest noted max heart rate at the end of a speed interval where I feel like I can't hold that pace any longer. Anytime that occurs, I note the new number, and I begin using the new, higher number as my max heart rate for calculations.

TWENTY MINUTE + FIVE TEST Perform your endurance activity at a comfortably hard pace for 20 minutes. Then switch to a fast pace, as if you were at the finish of a race. Hold that pace for five minutes, and then take your heart rate. If you start out too fast and can't make it to the end, stop and take your heart rate. **Do not push yourself to a point where you think you are even remotely close to passing out.**

Boosting Aerobic Capacity

If you want to build endurance and increase your speed, you need to increase your body's ability to transport and use oxygen during intense exercise. Aerobic capacity, also known as VO_2 max, is the maximal amount of oxygen your body can consume during maximal intensity exercise. The higher your VO_2 max, the better your body will be at creating energy.

There's a bunch of scientific stuff that I could share about how energy is created. If you're like most people, you'd skim over it and wouldn't be able to recall it tomorrow anyway. So I'm going to skip over all that and get right down to what you really need to know.

At this point, you might be wondering how it is possible to train for a long-distance event while training at a moderate pace. I've heard many runners claim that to race fast, you must train fast. And though it is true that some training needs to be at race pace, you'll want to incorporate a variety of moderate and high-intensity workouts throughout your training.

Types of Workouts You'll Include in Your Plan

I want to introduce you to three types of training: low-intensity steady state, fartlek, and high-intensity interval training.

LOW-INTENSITY STEADY STATE A low-intensity workout can be incorporated into the training plan frequently. The majority of research studies on endurance and high-intensity training consider anything below 75 percent of your max heart rate to be moderate- or low-intensity training.

FARTLEK *Fartlek* is Swedish for "speed play," which means this workout should be relaxed and fun. You can leave your watch or other technology at home because you'll complete the entire exercise by feel. Fartleks are a great transition between low-intensity steady-state work and high-intensity interval work. Remember that your body needs time to build up a tolerance for distance, repetitive movements, power, and high-intensity intervals. The fartlek is a safe workout that you can use to ease into high-intensity work. If you get injured often, or you're someone who puts a lot of pressure on yourself to hit certain paces, this can be a safe—and fun—way to get in some speed training.

Start out with an easy warm-up for 10 to 15 minutes. Then, for the remainder of the workout, vary your pace with no particular pattern or time in mind. This will work for running, cycling, walking, swimming, or any other endurance activity. When I'm working with runners, I will have them count lampposts or driveways and run hard for a certain number of them, then ease up for a certain number of them. You can also listen to music and run harder during the chorus. There are no rules other than to pick up the pace a few times throughout the workout, and to do so when you feel like it.

HIGH-INTENSITY INTERVAL TRAINING As I touched on in the heart rate training section, this is where the magic happens. A little bit of high-intensity interval training (HIIT) goes a long way. This is great news for people who want to increase their aerobic capacity while taking Dr. O'Keefe's research on heart health into consideration. For HIIT to be effective, you want your heart rate to be 85 to 95 percent of your max. This means you are working hard, and if you tried to talk, you could only get out one or two words at a time. A beginner athlete (or an athlete over 40 years old) would want one HIIT session a week, while an experienced athlete (or an athlete under 40) could do two or three HIIT sessions a week. Traditional higher-intensity workouts such as tempo runs, track work, and interval training fall into this category.

There is plenty of research supporting HIIT as a means of increasing VO_2 max in previously sedentary individuals and elite athletes. A study in the *International Journal of Environmental Research and Public Health* conducted by Bryant R. Byrd and colleagues showed that a combination of moderate-intensity continuous training, HIIT, and strength training elicited significantly greater improvements in VO_2 max than moderate-intensity continuous training alone. One hundred percent of the study participants saw an increase in VO_2 max with just one HIIT session plus strength training per week, in addition to the moderate-intensity exercise.

CAUTION:

High-intensity training is something you ease into. As you start incorporating long and short intervals, you will add a few minutes or a few intervals at a time.

Although HIIT has been shown to elicit comparable or superior improvements in cardiorespiratory fitness relative to moderate-intensity continuous exercise training, the American College of Sports Medicine recommends HIIT following an initial conditioning phase of two to three months.

Excessive high-intensity workouts can lead to elevated cortisol and could leave you hormonally depleted. Rest, recovery, and the addition of moderate-intensity exercise is recommended.

Introducing Polarized Training

You might have noticed a pattern here: I'm encouraging you to perform at two extremes—either at very high intensity or at very low intensity, with little exercise in the gray zone in between. This is referred to as polarized training, and there is substantial research to support its effectiveness for endurance athletes.

A study by Dr. Thomas Stöggl and Dr. Billy Sperlich published in *Frontiers in Physiology* showed that polarized training resulted in greater improvements to key endurance metrics in well-trained endurance athletes than high-intensity interval training, lactate threshold training, or high-volume training. To take advantage of polarized training, an athlete divides their training time in the following way:

* About 75 percent of the time in low- to moderate-intensity activity, with the heart rate below 75 percent of max.
* Around 5 percent of the time spent in the area we previously defined as the gray zone, with the heart rate at 75 to 85 percent of max.
* About 20 percent of training time in the high-intensity range, with the heart rate at about 85 to 95 percent of max.
  Math note: For an athlete who wants to adhere to Dr. O'Keefe's guideline of no more than two and a half hours of high-intensity exercise per week, 20 percent of a 12-hour training week is 2.4 hours.

BE GOOD ᴛᴏ YOURSELF

Reflect on your most peaceful moments of the past week. When did you feel most at ease and joyful? Is there a place you can go where you can feel the stress of the day melt away? Is there a person who always makes you smile? Does your heart flutter when your dog snuggles beside you? Does painting, writing, or playing a card game bring you delight? What do you look forward to? What makes your heart sing?

Gratitude is the key to living a healthy life. Research shows that a gratitude practice leads to increased happiness and feelings of peacefulness. Appreciating your surroundings, the people in your life, and the large and small moments that make up the day elevates mood, strengthens relationships, improves health, and even helps you sleep better.

As you reflect on the peaceful and joyful moments from your day, take the time to jot a few notes in your journal. Simply knowing this gratitude practice will become part of your routine causes you to become more aware of things that bring you joy. And that awareness magnifies all that is good in your life, ultimately sending more peace and joy your way.

The Importance of Rest and Recovery

No training discussion would be complete without a conversation about rest and recovery. As much as you love to train, it's not your full-time job, and it probably doesn't pay the bills. Instead, your training is squeezed into your day between your career, family, social obligations, and chores. And if you're lucky, you get six or seven hours of sleep each night.

The major difference between a professional athlete and a recreational athlete is that professional athletes are obsessive about recovery. When they are not training, they are engaged in active recovery, rest, or self-care.

* Active recovery could mean taking a walk or doing yoga.
* Rest could include sitting with your feet up, taking a nap, or making sure you get a minimum of seven hours of sleep each night.
* Self-care might be massage, meditation, foam rolling, or a steam treatment.

A training plan that incorporates proper rest and recovery should alternate hard days and easy days, giving the body time to recover from hard efforts. (There are exceptions to this, such as consecutive hard efforts like two days of medium-long runs back-to-back instead of one 20-mile run, as a way to gain training adaptations with a lower risk of injury.) The plan will also include a cutback week every three to five weeks, when the training volume is cut by 20 to 30 percent so the body gets additional rest.

Training adaptations do not occur while you exercise. They take place at rest. If you want to reap the benefits of your work, you must become serious about rest. Nutrition is also an important element in endurance training. Let's learn more about food and its role in your endurance training.

CHAPTER 3

FOOD

NUTRITION CAN BE a source of confusion for many people because there is no one best way to eat. There are a lot of opinions about it. Nutrition experts at the Harvard T. H. Chan School of Public Health created the Healthy Eating Plate to address the problems they saw in the US Department of Agriculture's MyPlate (which was created to complement the Food Pyramid), and the US Olympic Committee (USOC) created its own plate to help athletes make choices that will fuel their sports performance. Additionally, there are dozens of dietary approaches that flood the headlines with promises of health, fat loss, and chiseled abs.

As you read this chapter, I encourage you to take in all the information, prepare to make some incremental changes in your eating habits, and then observe what's working for your body. Using the RET approach, use a notebook to log your food and track how you feel. If you ever have concerns or want an expert to help you sort it all out, be sure to consult a registered dietitian.

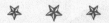

Eating for Power

If we are going to talk about getting the most out of the body we're living in, we need to talk about nutrition. For optimal health, peak brain function, and maximum athletic performance, our bodies need nutrient-dense, real foods. This isn't new information, but in the industrialized world—the United States in particular—sugar-filled, processed foods packed with ingredients we can't pronounce have become widely available. Product packaging is an art and science unto itself, featuring pictures of produce, farms, or beautiful scenery that help you associate the food item with nature. My advice: Look past the artwork and focus on the product's origin and ingredients list instead.

We all have days when time is short and we rely on convenience foods, but when eating out or choosing foods that come in a box becomes the norm, it's time to take a fresh look at our habits.

Food is fuel—not just for training and racing, but for our everyday lives. Food that fuels us is rich in phytochemicals, vitamins, minerals, healthy fats, and fiber. It is good for our brains, builds muscle, and gives us energy.

In contrast, a diet with an emphasis on processed foods and sugar increases our risk of obesity, metabolic syndrome, type 2 diabetes, heart disease, and some cancers. It also spikes our blood sugar, causing blood sugar crashes that leave us cranky and lethargic. Additionally, it contributes to inflammation that is linked to disease. Athletes should be aware that highly processed foods also limit the body's ability to adequately recover from workouts.

Food can be a loaded topic. There are those who believe foods should not be labeled "good" or "bad" because such classifications could lead to anxiety and possibly even disordered eating. An extreme obsession with maintaining a healthy diet is called orthorexia. Akin to anorexia, and sometimes occurring alongside it, orthorexia is marked by a highly limited diet, fear of eating the "wrong things," and general anxiety toward food. While orthorexia is fundamentally an anxiety disorder, according to The Body Project at Bradley University, athletes are at a higher risk for developing this condition. This may be due to the emphasis on food selection to enhance performance.

If you, your coach, or your peers are concerned that you might have developed an unhealthy obsession with food, which infringes on your quality of life or possibly causes you to cut back on calories and miss out on key nutrients, schedule an appointment with a therapist or registered dietitian specializing in eating disorders.

If we are going to apply the principles of responsive endurance training to how we fuel our bodies, not just for sports but so that we can live full, energetic, and joyful lives, we need to have compassion for ourselves when it comes to eating. That means we should do our best to eat foods that provide energy, fight disease, and keep inflammation at healthy levels. It also means that we should practice moderation, and if we want to socialize while refueling with donuts and coffee after a Saturday morning group run, we should do that, too, on occasion.

Ideally, the majority of what we eat would be real, whole foods—ingredients we can pick up at a farmers' market, meals with recognizable ingredients, and minimally processed foods that we prepare at home. I realize that's not always possible with work, entertaining, and super-busy weeknights—so no guilt trips here! Food is woven into every part of life, including how we celebrate. As an athlete trying to nourish your body, it can sometimes be a struggle when you're surrounded by people who don't share your appreciation for food as fuel.

The Big Picture

When we talk about nutrition, it's important to remember that everybody is different. Again, this is another reason to use your journal to track the details of your sleep, nutrition, exercise, and general well-being. As you replace processed and sugar-filled foods with nutrient-dense foods, you might notice some of the following things:

* Improved sleep
* Reduced pain
* Increased energy
* Less bloating and GI distress
* Brighter skin
* Diminished brain fog
* Enhanced ability to maintain a healthy body composition

Hero Foods

For optimal health and well-being, I recommend that the majority of the food you consume come in the form of fresh fruits, vegetables, protein, nuts and seeds, grains, dairy, and healthy fats. If you're looking for some hero foods—foods that pack a punch and support health and athletic performance—try adding some of these nutrient-dense foods to your diet:

QUINOA This ancient grain is gluten-free and loaded with protein, fiber, carbs, magnesium, and other essential nutrients. It's versatile and can be eaten with eggs for breakfast, mixed with oatmeal or chia seeds as a cereal, or used in place of rice in tacos or stuffed peppers. If you can't tell, it's one of my family's favorites.

SWEET POTATOES A slow-digesting carb providing beta-carotene, fiber, vitamins A and C, magnesium, potassium, and antioxidants, sweet potatoes should be at the top of every endurance athlete's list. Sweet potatoes can be consumed during endurance activities (if you want to carry real food), and they are beneficial when you're refueling after a workout (just add a bit of protein, and you have the perfect snack for replenishing glycogen and beginning the process of repairing your muscles!).

CHIA SEEDS First made famous in the 1970s with the Chia Pet, the chia seed became a favorite of runners after the release of *Born to Run* by Christopher McDougall. In the book, McDougall described the combination of chia seeds and water that the Tarahumara tribe uses to maintain energy and remain hydrated. Chia seeds have anti-inflammatory properties and help with muscle recovery. They are loaded with fiber, protein, fat, calcium, manganese, magnesium, and phosphorus. Check out my Chia Pudding recipe in this book (see page 126).

SALMON Omega-3 fatty acids, abundant in salmon, support heart health and reduce inflammation, making this protein-packed food ideal for athletes. Your doctor might have suggested taking fish oil capsules for your heart, your brain, or your bones. Salmon is a great way to get this nutrient, and it's delicious for breakfast, lunch, or dinner.

EGGS Once eggs were demonized because the yolks are high in cholesterol, but we now know that this nutritional powerhouse with 6 grams of protein helps raise our HDL (good cholesterol) while also helping lower our triglycerides. They provide lutein and zeaxanthin, powerful antioxidants known for protecting the body from free radicals, which contribute to disease and inflammation. Packed with 13 vitamins and minerals, eggs add nutritional variety. Bonus: They are also considered an antiaging superfood.

BLUEBERRIES A recent study in the *American Journal of Clinical Nutrition* showed that eating a cup of blueberries a day reduced the risk of cardiovascular disease by up to 15 percent. Rich in anthocyanins, the nutrient that gives fruits and vegetables their purple color, blueberries may benefit cardiovascular health, enhance memory, and aid in muscle recovery after a workout. Tip: In many cases, frozen fruits and veggies contain more nutrients than fresh ones (due to the harvesting and shipping timelines), so don't shy away from frozen berries, especially in the winter months when it's more difficult to buy fresh, local fruit.

BANANAS No list of hero foods for endurance athletes would be complete without mention of bananas. After all, bananas are the most popular postrace food on the planet! Bananas are easy to digest, making them an ideal food to eat before, during, and after a race. This popular source of potassium comes in its own packaging, so it's also convenient for snacking when you're on the go. Green bananas contain resistant starch, which provides the food for good bacteria in the gut.

* Broccoli
* Green tea
* Kale
* Low-sugar yogurt listing lactobacillus acidophilus on the label
* Oatmeal
* Pickles
* Pumpkin
* Sauerkraut
* Spinach
* Walnuts and almonds

Food Flops

By now, you're probably getting a good idea about the types of foods that work against your body when it comes to recovery, inflammation, and energy stores. You'll want to limit or avoid processed and packaged foods, treats and drinks with added sugars, snacks like chips and cookies, and items with additives and dyes.

A study published on *BMJ Open* on the effects of ultra-processed foods and added sugars in the diet showed that ultra-processed foods contribute almost 60 percent of calories and 90 percent of added sugars consumed in the United States. The high consumption of added sugars is associated with obesity, type 2 diabetes, elevated lipids in the blood, hypertension, and coronary heart disease, all of which we also see increase when developing countries adopt a Western diet.

You know this stuff has a negative effect on your health. The question is, what are you going to do about it? Again, moderation is key. I'm not suggesting that you need to give up all these foods for life. Just consume them sparingly, and fill your plate with nutrient-dense fruits, vegetables, nuts, seeds, and grains.

A registered dietitian can help you fine-tune your nutrition, but to get started, here are some food flops that will be on any reputable dietitian's list:

I'm clumping these together because they are filled with chemicals, dyes, and sugars. These drinks often contain high fructose corn syrup, contribute to inflammation, are linked to obesity, and are generally bad for your teeth and bones. If I could recommend only one dietary change that will contribute to better health, it would be eliminating sugar-filled drinks.

ARTIFICIAL SWEETENERS In case you thought you found a loophole that would allow you to continue consuming sweet drinks, guess again.

According to the *Harvard Health Publishing* blog, the Food and Drug Administration (FDA) has approved five artificial sweeteners: saccharin, acesulfame, aspartame, neotame, and sucralose, in addition to the natural low-calorie sweetener stevia. However, the FDA's approval doesn't mean that all artificial sweeteners are good for us.

A study posted on the American Diabetes Association website shows that daily diet soda consumption is associated with a 36 percent greater relative risk of metabolic syndrome and a 67 percent greater relative risk of type 2 diabetes compared with nonconsumption. In addition, in a study where rats were exposed to water sweetened with saccharin and intravenous cocaine, 94 percent preferred the saccharin over cocaine, which is known to be highly addictive.

There is limited research on stevia, which may be safe for most populations. However, we do not know how stevia affects gut health, metabolism, or immunity. While it is considered safe, there is not much research on its safety during pregnancy or for consumption by children. It's also important to note that some packaged stevia products are blends that could spike blood sugar.

SUGARS One last word about sugar. Added sugar is hiding in 74 percent of packaged foods, according to SugarScience, a website developed by a team of health scientists at the University of California, San Francisco. The majority of Americans have gotten the message that high fructose corn syrup is bad for health, so now manufacturers have begun hiding sugar on labels by using a variety of names. The SugarScience site lists 61 different names for sugar, including sucrose, barley malt, dextrose, maltose, rice syrup, beet sugar, brown sugar, cane juice, honey, agave nectar, and coconut sugar.

Here is a list of other foods to avoid, or to eat in moderation—after reading the label and considering the nutritional impact:

WHITE BREAD Replace white bread with whole-grain bread, or consider going without bread and substituting a food from the hero food list.

CHIPS AND FRIES If you love the crunchy taste of chips, try making your own by dehydrating potatoes in a food dehydrator. You can prepare your own fries by slicing a superfood (like sweet potatoes), drizzling them with avocado oil, and baking them.

PASTRIES, COOKIES, CAKES, AND CANDIES There's just no good substitute for these treats. Consume them in moderation, and eat fruits, nuts, and berries when you feel the urge to snack.

FOODS LABELED "LOW FAT" OR "GLUTEN-FREE" Don't be tricked into thinking these foods are automatically good for you. A review of the label will usually show that the manufacturer has added sugar and lots of artificial ingredients to make them taste appealing. Remember that whenever you're eating packaged, premade, processed food, it was made by someone intent on selling a product and not necessarily on giving you healthy food.

FAST FOOD Some fast foods are better than others, and not everything on a fast-food restaurant's menu is completely lacking in nutritional value. Many restaurants now offer select menus to appeal to health-conscious consumers. Keep an eye on portion sizes, be on the lookout for sugars in ketchup and dressings, and stick with the least-processed options available.

Protein versus Carbs versus Fat

High carb. Low fat. High fat. Low carb. Paleo. Whole 30. Keto. Mediterranean. Standard American Diet. Vegetarian. Vegan. There are so many ways of eating, and everyone insists their method is best. How does an endurance athlete begin to figure out which approach to take?

First, let's go back to the principles of responsive endurance training. Each body is different: Therefore, it is important to record your meals in your journal and take time to reflect on your diet and how your body responds to it. As you begin to eat more fresh, unprocessed, nutrient-dense food, what do you notice about how you think, feel, and perform? Use what you observe to choose foods that energize you and keep your brain feeling sharp.

What Are the Roles of Carbs, Protein, and Fat in the Athlete's Diet?

CARBS Carbohydrates have gotten a bad rap amid a surge of enthusiasm for low-carb, high-fat diets. It's important to remember that quality carbohydrates are required for a variety of bodily functions, and carbs are necessary for the creation of glycogen, which is what our bodies use for energy when we shift into higher-intensity efforts. By avoiding carbs, an athlete risks missing out on the critical nutrients found only in carbs.

However, not all carbs are created equal, and it's important to choose a variety of carbohydrate sources to make sure you get the nutrients your body needs. I could eat a candy bar with 29 grams of carbs, with 20 grams coming from sugar. Or I could choose a cup of sweet potato totaling 27 grams of carbs and also get potassium, fiber, protein, vitamin A, calcium, vitamin C, iron, vitamin B6, and magnesium. When choosing foods, it's not just about calories or carbs. The nutritional quality of the food matters.

PROTEIN Protein is critical for muscle recovery and growth. Your hard work goes to waste if you do not provide your body with enough protein to repair muscles. When you hear people talk about branched-chain amino acids (BCAAs), they are referring to a type of amino acid found in protein-rich food sources. It's not necessary to rely on protein shakes and BCAA supplements to get the protein your body requires for maximum athletic performance. You can get all you need by consuming a variety of plant or animal proteins such as meat, fish, eggs, cheese, and beans.

FAT Fats can be confusing because for decades we were told that fats cause heart disease and should be avoided. Concerned about their health, consumers switched to margarines and chose low-fat foods. It wasn't until recently that a variety of health and nutrition organizations changed their stance on fat. It is now acknowledged that healthy fats are an important energy source required for helping the body absorb fat-soluble vitamins. Some healthy fat sources include avocado, chia seeds, fatty fish (like salmon), coconut oil, avocado oil, olive oil, and nuts. Dietary fat can be used as an energy source, and the omega-3s found in healthy fats help reduce inflammation, which is necessary as your body recovers after exercise.

To gain clarity on sports nutrition, I spoke with Rebecca McConville, a nutrition and performance expert, registered dietitian, and board-certified sports specialist. She encourages a customized and balanced approach to nutrition and is the author of *Finding Your Sweet Spot*, a book that teaches athletes how to optimize their energy balance. She recommended the Athlete's Plates, which are a collaboration between the United States Olympic Committee's sport dietitians and the University of Colorado at Colorado Springs' Sport Nutrition Graduate Program. From the nutrition section of the Team USA website, athletes can download worksheets that provide guidelines for how to eat on easy, moderate, and hard training days.

On moderate training days, protein should fill one-quarter of the plate. A serving size of protein is about the size of the palm of your hand. The remainder of the plate should be equally split between grains and produce served with a healthy fat, each taking up half of the three-quarters of the plate that remains after protein fills the first quarter of the plate. For reference, visit www.teamusa.org/nutrition.

In using the Athlete's Plates, Rebecca recommends that athletes eat a different grain for breakfast, lunch, and dinner and that they have at least four grains in rotation throughout the week. For produce, she says we should aim for two or three different colors per meal, plus a source of fat to help with nutrient absorption.

Rebecca adds that there's no cookie-cutter approach, and each person needs to be attuned to what works for them. She reminds us that we need carbs for daily functions. "On every given day," she says, "we need carbs to provide fuel to our brain. We need carbs for fiber. We need carbs to create and support our neurotransmitters, to sleep, to think, and to enhance our immune system. Carbs suppress cortisol, and so carbs enhance the immune system. We want our glycogen over time to increase; that's how we are able to run longer and faster and stay hydrated. Carbs reduce the risk of injury by decreasing inflammation."

Dr. Mark Cucuzzella, founder of Healthy Running Medical Education, a biomechanics expert, and a professor at West Virginia University School of Medicine, agrees that there's not one prescriptive way of eating. He says we need to look at the individual and take their overall health into consideration when determining the ratio of carbohydrates, fats, and protein. He gives the example of someone whose doctor has suggested they train for a 5K because of a health scare. If that person has type 2 diabetes or is prediabetic, a high-carb diet is not going to improve that person's health because their body is intolerant to carbohydrates. Instead, a person in this situation would want to reduce their carbohydrate intake and consume a higher percentage of fat and protein.

However, a metabolically healthy athlete who can tolerate carbohydrates should not be afraid to consume a plate of pasta or slices of whole-grain bread. Cucuzzella says, "If you eat carbs, you burn carbs. If you eat fat, you burn fat. Most of the Kenyan elite marathoners eat 600 to 900 grams a day of carbohydrates. They are not diabetic. They are not insulin resistant. They can eat that way. But they aren't eating white bread. The smartest athletes are eating real-food carbohydrates—beans, lentils—if you don't have an issue with flours, you can have some whole-grain bread."

A person whose blood sugar is not in a normal range, or who is gaining weight in their midsection, might want to consult their physician or work with a dietitian to find a balance of carbs, protein, and fats that improves their metabolic health.

Creating a Custom Nutrition Plan

If the idea of a custom approach to nutrition piques your interest, you'll also want to explore nutrigenomics. This relatively new field of study looks at the relationship between nutrition and genetics, allowing individuals to create a customized approach to nutrition. Research originally published in *Frontiers in Nutrition* says that genetic differences are known to impact absorption, metabolism, uptake, utilization and excretion of nutrients, and food bioactives.

There are a variety of commercial tests that will provide nutrition recommendations based on your genetic profile; however, if you take this route, you must also be prepared for the possibility of finding out you have a genetic variant for certain diseases. In addition to providing information on how your body absorbs micronutrients, you could discover you have the potential to develop celiac disease, that you carry the BRCA breast cancer genes, that you are lactose intolerant, or that you are likely to be sensitive to caffeine.

Working with a registered dietitian, you can take a personalized approach to nutrition that considers your athletic goals, any nutrient deficiencies you currently have, and any food allergies or sensitivities you have. A sports dietitian or nutritionist can help you dial in your nutrition and customize a plan.

CAFFEINE AND SPORTS DRINKS: FRENEMIES?

Caffeine is widely used across all segments of society, and in the world of sports, caffeine is considered to be a performance-enhancing drug. It's legal, but is it good for us? As with many elements of nutrition, it depends.

Caffeine is a stimulant that can increase reaction time, delay the perception of fatigue, and lessen sensations of exertion and pain. Students and drivers appreciate caffeine for its ability to positively affect cognitive function and alertness. According to the US Olympic Committee's sport nutrition team, caffeine can improve endurance and short-term, high-intensity sport performance.

The USOC lists these possible side effects of caffeine: anxiety, overstimulation, jitteriness, mental confusion, elevated resting heart rate, restlessness, inability to focus, gastric irritation, mild diuretic effect, insomnia, and addiction. It's also important to note that caffeine is not recommended during pregnancy, and it can affect fertility in addition to raising cortisol levels and possibly taxing the adrenal glands. Each person reacts differently to caffeine, and it may affect your sleep, which is also a necessary part of recovery.

If you choose to use caffeine to enhance your training and athletic performance, you should know that the FDA recommends a maximum intake of 400 milligrams, or two to three cups of coffee, a day. The USOC does not recommend the use of energy drinks because they have the potential to contain banned substances. And you should never consume energy drinks with alcohol because the combination can be lethal.

Because I'm a fan of consuming real food, I encourage you to consider what other ingredients are present in your caffeine source. "Sports drinks"—a term chosen quite deliberately for branding purposes—often contain preservatives, dyes, artificial sweeteners, and other chemicals that may or may not be safe for long-term consumption. Manufacturers of these beverages have spent a great deal of marketing dollars sponsoring extreme sporting events or creating marketing campaigns that feature famous athletes. This suggests to the buyer that the beverage itself was designed for athleticism or physical performance. The ingredients list tells a different story. Caffeinated beverages in the form of coffee and soft drinks often include sugars and artificial sweeteners that can cause inflammation, which wreaks havoc on the body.

When it comes to caffeine consumption, this is another case for reading the label, being aware of what you are putting into your body, and using your journal to track how your body reacts to what you consume.

Blood Sugar Mastery

The last time you went to the doctor, how much time did anyone spend talking to you about nutrition? Nutrition and lifestyle factors contribute to the four leading causes of death in the United States, yet only one-fifth of medical schools require students to take a nutrition course.

Food is medicine, and we look to our doctors for wellness education, but most are not adequately trained to educate their patients about nutrition. I believe these facts shine a light on some of the challenges present in our health care system. Because of their training, our doctors are more likely to prescribe anti-inflammatory pills and pain relievers to address pain and inflammation than to suggest that we examine our food choices. Many doctors will prescribe statins and blood pressure medications, rather than suggesting dietary adjustments and exercise. Furthermore, exercise, meditation, and nutrition are rarely mentioned when doctors are addressing the many medical conditions these interventions can improve.

I don't mean to sound conspiratorial or to deny the many accomplishments and treatment advancements of modern medicine. However, many of the food products available to us in stores are not produced in our best interest, and for the most part, our doctors are not trained to provide quality nutrition counseling.

To further complicate things, major food brands often provide research funding for studies that show their products do not have negative consequences for health, and lobbyists for consumer products invest major funds to influence regulatory bodies.

We've become a society that expects quick fixes. We need to stop taking the easy way out. We need to be prepared to do the hard work necessary to make long-term changes that affect our health. This starts with doing the research and advocating for ourselves.

Now that I've provided a little background, I'll get off my soapbox and share some information about why nutrition is especially important for endurance athletes. The big picture: The foods you choose affect energy and recovery.

Added Sugars and Their Role in Inflammation

The biggest source of added sugar in the diet is sweetened drinks, but even if you steer clear of sugary drinks, you're probably consuming sugar you didn't even know was in your food. It's hidden in cereals, ketchup, pasta sauce, yogurt, granola, dried fruit, and many foods you might consider "healthy."

Why is this important to athletes? Because inflammation causes pain. And if you are constantly feeding your body sugar, which causes chronic inflammation, your body cannot adequately recover from your training efforts. If you want to give your body every advantage to heal so that you get the most out of each workout, limit foods that create an inflammatory response.

Overconsumption of sugar also impairs mitochondria and can cause nutrient depletion. By choosing foods with higher sugar content, we are choosing fewer nutrient-dense foods. Foods loaded with sugar deplete the body of important nutrients such as vitamin D, calcium, magnesium, chromium, and vitamin C. For your body to function its best, it needs the nutrients present in real food.

Inflammation, when it works as intended, is the body's way of protecting itself. Acute inflammation is the immune system's protective reaction to stimuli that it believes are harmful, and it is desirable when we have a scrape, cut, or virus. Inflammation is also our body's way of providing a healing response after a workout as it seeks to repair tissues. When inflammation works properly, it is protective and beneficial. It's part of the process that repairs the muscle fibers after exercise so our muscles become stronger.

When it becomes chronic, inflammation is bad for our health. Uncontrolled inflammation plays a role in heart disease, stroke, dementia, depression, accelerated aging, and type 2 diabetes. Lifestyle factors such as chronic stress, an excessively sugary diet, and excessive exercise can contribute to inflammation that is not helpful.

If you work with a health professional, they can look for signs of chronic inflammation with some blood tests. Physicians can measure C-reactive protein and homocysteine levels, both of which indicate inflammation in the body, and look at red blood cell damage with an HbA1C test measuring blood sugar.

How Do We Manage Inflammation and Keep It in Check?

Clearly, diet has an impact on inflammation. Earlier in this chapter, we looked at some of the foods that can have an inflammatory effect on the body. Sugar plays a significant role in inflammation, and unfortunately sugar can be addictive. One of the reasons we crave sugar is because it can give us a quick energy boost. Carbohydrates that are high on the glycemic index can cause blood sugar to spike. When blood sugar crashes, it can leave us feeling lethargic or drained of energy. To compensate, we reach for another food that provides a quick release of sugar, and the cycle begins again.

If you've ever reached for a candy bar for quick energy when you can't focus after lunch, you're locked into this cycle in which your food choices are creating peaks and valleys in your blood sugar. You're better off choosing foods that keep blood sugar in the normal range, thus avoiding blood sugar spikes. You really can't go wrong with a snack that includes fresh fruits and vegetables, along with a bit of protein.

Signs of chronic inflammation include depression, anxiety, pain, fatigue, digestive issues, and brain fog. If you have an injury that is slow to heal, or you do not recover from workouts as expected, these could also be signs that your body has chronic inflammation.

Ways to Reduce Inflammation

* The average American consumes 17 teaspoons of added sugar each day. One of the best ways to reduce inflammation is to decrease consumption of foods with obvious added sugars, such as candy, cookies, and pastries.
* Sugar is in 74 percent of packaged foods in the United States. Adding fresh foods, cooking from scratch, and cutting back on packaged foods will help you reduce your sugar intake.
* A 20-minute session of moderate-intensity exercise is enough to create an anti-inflammatory response in the body. This is good news for people who have medical conditions in which inflammation plays a role.
* The body responds to stress by creating inflammation, and we are learning that mindfulness techniques like meditation can influence inflammation, immunity, and aging.

Lack of proper nutrition can affect athletic performance. You must fuel your body with nutrient-dense foods to perform your best. Will one glass of wine or one piece of cake hurt? Probably not. I'm not asking you to live without foods and beverages that enhance your happiness or improve your life. It's when we cross over into chronic or excessive behaviors that most things— whether it's exercise or the foods we consume—become a problem.

ALCOHOL AND THE ATHLETE

Will participating in your running club's beer mile have a long-term effect on your training? What about an occasional glass of wine? As with any choice you make with your training and nutrition, it's important to weigh the risks and rewards of the behavior. An occasional drink probably won't hurt you; however, if popping open a beer is a regular occurrence, you might want to consider the timing. According to the USOC Sports Nutrition Alcohol Factsheet, there is no beneficial effect of alcohol on athletic performance, and it is best to avoid alcohol within 48 hours of training or competition.

There are many reasons why alcohol impairs athletic performance—and not much science supporting its use. If you enjoy a glass of wine on a Saturday night after your long run, you should know that alcohol affects the quality of sleep, which is a necessary part of the recovery process. Alcohol impairs coordination and reaction time and, in addition to raising your heart rate, will make that workout seem harder than it actually is. Athletes who drink are 30 percent more likely to get a musculoskeletal injury compared to athletes who abstain. Research also shows that alcohol consumption can impair recovery after a workout, and alcohol inhibits the body's ability to absorb nutrients. It's important to remember that alcohol is a diuretic, so if you do imbibe, remember to hydrate well before your next training session.

The best advice is to abstain from drinking or to consume alcohol in moderation. Both the National Collegiate Athletic Association and the USOC provide useful information regarding alcohol consumption (see the Resources section).

Training Period Meal Plan

It would be wonderful if I could give you a formula created for you and you alone detailing exactly what you should eat and when. I'm sure you're seeing a pattern by now. Each body is different, and there is no one-size-fits-all solution. How you eat for peak performance will differ from what works best for your training partner. The most important consideration is whether your dietary habits are putting you on the path to success. The best way to determine this is to use responsive endurance training to track what you're eating and to note how you feel before, during, and after each workout.

If grocery carts, drive-through lines, and Instagram party pictures are any indication, most of us have never gone through an extended period when we've given up highly processed, sugar-filled, inflammatory foods. My first recommendation is always to take the time to address your dietary weaknesses. I challenge you to devote at least three weeks to improving your nutrition habits. If you are like most people who have taken this approach, you will notice a difference in how you feel, and you will probably discover at least one food that is not your friend.

Your nutrition needs vary depending on your activity levels. As you learned earlier in the chapter, the USOC Athlete's Plates are a good place to start when learning how to balance carbs, protein, and fats. They have diet recommendations for days when the intensity of your activity is easy, moderate, and hard. The balance of carbs from grains versus fruits and vegetables changes depending on your activity level. Protein boosts metabolism and is required to repair and build muscle. We all need protein, so don't shortchange yourself here.

Many athletes believe there is a benefit to training on an empty stomach. While you can certainly test that theory, there are exercise physiologists who believe a properly fueled workout is more

WHY WE RACE
ATHLETICISM AND AGING GRACEFULLY

What does Sharon Doerre, a 52-year-old mother of three, have in common with Teddy Roosevelt, Bradley Cooper, Bram Stoker, Hugh Laurie, and Stephen Hawking? Rowing!

Sharon first became interested in rowing in her late 40s when she couldn't make sense of her daughter's rowing practices. Her journey began as she perused the internet to improve her knowledge, learning the difference between sweeping and sculling, studying boat configurations, and figuring out the rules.

It takes tremendous physical conditioning to row, which means that rowers must put in a considerable amount of work outside the boat. The first summer Sharon's daughter moved to the varsity team, Sharon decided to keep her company during workouts. They ran and cycled together. By the end of the summer, Sharon had a desire to become more competitive with her workouts.

Soon after, Sharon began using an indoor rowing machine. She was inspired by an article about a 70-year-old Dutch woman who set a new world rowing record in the 70 to 74 age division. Sharon set a goal of hitting that world record time (for women 20 years older than she was)—and she's currently less than nine seconds away from that time, rowing in the 90th percentile for her own age division.

Eventually, Sharon's daughter encouraged her to row on the water. When she turned 50, she set two goals: to run a 10K and to learn to row on the water. She took a "learn to row" class, which was two hours each Saturday and Sunday for three weeks—and has never looked back.

As she's become more serious about the sport, Sharon has dialed in her hydration and nutrition. She's also discovered that journaling is critical to her improvement as an athlete. The first thing she does when she returns home after a row is write in her journal. Some of the things she tracks include her weight that day, her hydration and enthusiasm, whether it was a morning or evening practice, who the coach was, the type of boat she was in, which oars she used, what she did well, what she needs to work on, and any cues the coach gave. She says there's often a gap between the words the coach uses to get a rower to make a physical pattern change and how her own body moves when she's trying to apply that feedback. She's found journaling to be helpful, because if she can't execute a movement properly on a particular day, she can often return to her notes and apply the feedback she was given as she develops new skills and gains experience.

As she's become more competitive, she's tailored her nutrition to help her maximize her potential. She says she doesn't drink soda or alcohol, eats fish one or two times a week, and consumes plenty of whole fruits and vegetables. She also weighs 30 pounds less than she did four years ago. Rowing burns a lot of calories, so Sharon pays close attention to her nutrition to make sure she has the calories to fuel her activity—and to avoid losing additional weight.

Not long ago, Sharon expressed an interest in joining a competitive team. Although she'd been rowing on the water for less than two years, she landed a spot on the team and participated in her first regatta in October 2019. She jumped right into the world of competitive rowing in a big way, participating in the Head of the Charles, the world's largest two-day rowing event, which attracts 11,000 athletes annually.

Sharon is a shining example of how responsive endurance training can help an athlete continue to improve performance and accept new challenges at any age.

effective. It makes sense to give your body the fuel it needs to perform so that each training session is a quality session. It doesn't take much food to give your body what it needs. A banana with peanut butter or another low-fat, low-fiber source of quality carbohydrates with a bit of protein will do. Other favorites include peanut butter on toast and oatmeal with nuts. But test the food you choose before race day, because not everyone can tolerate the same foods. For example, oatmeal could be more substantial than your body can digest while exercising. Digestion time also varies from person to person.

After your workout, shoot for a 3:1 or 4:1 ratio of carbs to protein within 30 minutes of exercising. This doesn't need to be a huge meal; 30 to 40 grams of carbs and 10 grams of protein will do. You could try three-quarters of a cup of quinoa or half a sweet potato with an egg on top, or chicken and roasted vegetables. If you are eating a meal within an hour of working out, you do not need to eat a post-workout snack, especially if you are trying to lose weight, or if your workout was lower in intensity.

BE GOOD ᴛᴏ YOURSELF

There is nothing more important than mind-set when it comes to getting the most out of your athletic ability. The thoughts you repeat to yourself become your reality, and they dictate your behavior. What you think—how you frame the events in your life—determines whether you sit on the sidelines and let life happen to you, or whether you leap out of bed each day and take charge.

When I started my podcast, *Power Up Your Performance*, I wanted to explore the champion's mind-set. I wanted to know what sets high achievers apart from others. One of the most noteworthy traits is that those who achieve greatness in sport and business treat themselves with compassion. They embrace the person they are today, and when they stumble, they extend the same grace to themselves as they would to a friend who struggles.

We are human. We make mistakes, and we need to be kind to ourselves so we have the courage to start again, as many times as it takes.

Top performers believe the world is full of possibilities, and they know that a positive mind-set is critical to success. It's this belief that we aren't defined by our setbacks, that we have the ability to create the life we desire, that drives high achievers.

Take time this week to recount your accomplishments and give yourself credit for all you've achieved and created in your life. Use compassion and positive self-talk to protect your resilience. YOU are remarkable and can do anything you set your mind to.

CHAPTER 4

BUILD YOUR
FOUNDATION

NOW, LET'S TAKE A LOOK at some of the ways that we should tailor training and fueling based on biological and physiological differences between various body types, as well as gender differences. We'll examine body types as another way of understanding how athletes can approach individualized training, and we'll explore relative energy deficiency in sport (RED-S), a syndrome that results from an imbalance between fueling and energy needs. Throughout this chapter, you'll see that there truly is a great deal of variability among bodies, and there's no one-size-fits-all approach. Men are not just hairy women, and women aren't just smaller men.

As you are exposed to more ideas, you'll gain insight that will help you discover what works for your body. Take notes as you move through the chapter. Does the information provide any insight that will help you become more resilient?

Body-Type Awareness

Each body is different, and that's a good thing! It's important to accept our bodies and celebrate what they can do at each stage of life. If we make time to care for our bodies, we will find that, even with setbacks, we are able to maximize our potential at every stage. I believe that all bodies are able to enjoy endurance sports, and we should focus less on how we look and more on taking the steps we can to get the most out of what we have in any given moment. A mother of a six-month-old will have very different concerns than the woman who is going through menopause or the middle-aged man who sits at a desk all day. Your body is made for movement, so don't let anyone's perception of what an endurance athlete looks like keep you from pursuing your athletic goals.

A somatotype is a way of classifying body types based on physical characteristics. There are three somatotypes, which are classifications doctors and trainers use to tailor nutrition and fitness plans.

ECTOMORPH An ectomorph is the long, lanky type who does not have much fat or muscle. When we think of the stereotypical basketball player or ballet dancer, this is the look that most often comes to mind. Ectomorphs have difficulty gaining both fat and muscle. Michael Phelps and Misty Copeland are ectomorphs.

MESOMORPH A mesomorph builds muscle easily and does not store much fat. Male mesomorphs have wider shoulders and a smaller waist, while female mesomorphs have the classic hourglass shape. This type is more likely to be naturally athletic. Arnold Schwarzenegger and Serena Williams are mesomorphs.

ENDOMORPH Endomorphs are sometimes referred to as big boned. They are more likely to store fat, and they gain weight easily. This body type is softer and curvier. Movement and a focus on nutrition are important for endomorphs. Amy Schumer and Jack Black are endomorphs.

Body Type	Nutrition Focus	Fitness Focus
Ectomorph	Consume protein to support muscle growth. Add at least 500 daily calories if the goal is to gain weight or muscle.	Excels at endurance. For increased muscle mass, cut back on cardio and focus on power and resistance to build strength.
Mesomorph	Higher calorie needs than other body types, due to bigger ratio of muscle mass. Divide the plate into thirds: carbohydrates, grains, and protein.	Excels at sports requiring power and speed. Include HIIT, strength training, steady-state (moderate-intensity) cardio, and plyometrics (see page 85).
Endomorph	Increase protein to build muscle mass, and include a blend of carbs and fats. If the goal is to gain lean muscle mass and lose fat, consume protein and quality fats, and limit carbs.	Struggles to maintain a lower body fat percentage. Increase movement throughout the day, and add resistance training to increase muscle mass and metabolism. Include high-intensity metabolic training techniques and moderate-intensity cardio.

In addition, a person can be a combination of two types. An ecto-endomorph's body has a pear shape, and the endo-ectomorph's body is apple shaped.

Knowing your somatotype can help you consider your nutrition and exercise strategies when it comes to building muscle and changing body composition.

Each body type requires a slightly different nutrition and fitness focus, according to articles on the National Academy of Sports Medicine and the American Council on Exercise websites.

This is just an introduction to nutrition and training for your body type. I highly recommend you read Dr. Stacy Sims's book, *ROAR*. Women especially will find this book beneficial, as it delves deep into eating and fueling strategies that take women's health and hormones into account.

Gender Variations

The field of gender-specific medicine is relatively new, but it has taught us that the biological and physiological differences between males and females affect every area of health. Prevention and treatment protocols for cardiovascular disease, diabetes, mood disorders, osteoporosis, cancer, and more are improved when gender is taken into account.

But what does gender-specific medicine have to do with endurance? This growing field tells us that we have only begun to understand how gender affects our health and athletic abilities. By becoming aware of some of the areas that affect performance, you have the power to make smart training decisions that will help you maximize your potential.

The best training advice will always be to listen to your body, so the following considerations will help you know what to look out for.

VO$_2$ Max

The biggest gender difference is that men typically have a higher VO$_2$ max. This measure of the body's ability to consume oxygen and convert it to energy during intense exercise is influenced by the size of the heart and lungs, how much muscle is present in the body, and hemoglobin levels, which all vary by sex.

Hormones

Testosterone and estrogen also affect athletic performance. Men and women have both hormones but in very different quantities. Testosterone contributes to muscle growth for both genders. With naturally lower testosterone levels, a woman can get stronger, but she will not easily build the bulky muscles we associate with males.

Estrogen affects body composition, strength, speed, and metabolism. At different stages in her life, a woman will experience changes in athletic performance based on the fluctuations of female hormones. It is important for female athletes who have not yet entered menopause to have periods, because missing periods is considered a sign that something is off in the balance of training, nutrition, and recovery. In menopause, a woman might notice a change in body composition that includes an accumulation of fat around her midsection, along with a reduced ability to efficiently cool herself when her body heats up during training.

Women may also notice changes in performance at different stages of their monthly cycle. This is a newer area of research, but there is evidence to support that women have improved performance during their period, while they may feel less energetic during ovulation.

Injury Risk

The Q angle is a measurement of the angle between the quadriceps muscles and the patellar tendon, and this is significant when it comes to knee injuries in female athletes. Women have a larger

Q angle than men because they have a wider pelvis. This essentially means women are more prone to knee injuries because of the way their quads pull on the kneecap.

Nutrition for Female Athletes

Dr. Stacy Sims, author of *ROAR: How to Match Your Food and Fitness to Your Female Physiology for Optimum Performance, Great Health, and a Strong, Lean Body for Life*, has a body of research relating to women's physiology. Her research is well documented in her book, and also in interviews and podcasts available online. *ROAR* is a fascinating look into the differences between men and women and how those differences should affect our nutrition and training. One of those differences relates to the hormone fluctuations women experience throughout their menstrual cycles.

A few days before her period, a woman is in a high-hormone phase. During this phase, it is harder to build muscle, hit high intensities, remain hydrated, and recover. In the low-hormone phase, which is during her period and the follicular phase, it is easier to race and build muscle.

Dr. Sims says we can use this information to tailor our nutrition to our menstrual cycles. During the high-hormone phase, women should focus on hydration, adding watery fruits and vegetables to increase blood volume. It's also important to consume additional protein during this phase to prevent the breakdown of muscle tissue. Most women are surprised to learn that their performance during their period is enhanced.

Women in menopause can also make nutritional adjustments. They become more intolerant to carbs and fructose, have a harder time cooling during exercise, encounter an inhibited ability to burn fat, and experience difficulty gaining muscle mass. In addition to practicing regular weight training to increase muscle mass, women in menopause should consume quality carbohydrates, focus on gut health and hydration, and consume protein.

What Do We Do with This Information?

Through training, we challenge the body to become stronger by adapting to the training stress we put it under. You should listen to your body, work with your coach, and consult medical professionals throughout the process.

* Work with your doctor to monitor iron levels and make supplement or nutrition adjustments as needed.
* Include resistance training to build muscle, which will transport more oxygen through the body while you're competing, while also making you stronger and less prone to injury.
* Consult with a coach who can help you analyze and address deficiencies with your biomechanics. Efficient running form can make up for the effects of a lower VO_2 max.
* Include interval training and HIIT workouts to boost endurance and speed.
* Remember that rest days help reduce cortisol and are just as important to building strength, speed, and endurance as hard training days.
* Keep a journal that tracks training activities, as well as details about your menstrual cycle (ovulation, start of period, energy levels). Note if you lose your period, and work with your doctor to make appropriate changes to your nutrition and training in order to restart it.

WHY WE RACE
BODY AND MIND WELLNESS

Missy Boser recalls returning from a vacation with her husband in 2012, looking at the vacation photos, and being shocked because she had not realized how big she had gotten. She decided to take control of how she looked and felt, and began a wellness journey that continues today. Initially, the focus was on nutrition, and she slowly added more movement into her life. On January 1, 2013, she ran her first 5K in freezing Minnesota temperatures. She remembers feeling exhilarated and knew her life would be forever changed.

Missy experiences anxiety and depression, but she quickly noticed that running made her feel better. As she did more endurance training, she realized running energized her—and that the longer she ran, the longer the effects lasted. She says that a 10-mile run makes her feel better for an entire day, and the effects of a three-mile run last for an afternoon. While she is careful to avoid overtraining, running plays an important part in managing her mental health. Many studies show that running can have as much of an impact on anxiety and depression as many medications do, and this is true for her. She adds that running boosts her confidence and reminds her she's capable of doing hard things, which also helps her manage anxiety symptoms.

Missy is a Girls on the Run Ambassador, and she has recently become a running coach. She explains that she wanted to become a coach because a number of medical and fitness professionals treated her like she was "less than" because of her weight. "I have gotten so much from running. I am not what most people think of when they think of a runner," she says. "I'm bigger, and someone who is bigger may feel more comfortable working with me because they know I'm not going to judge them."

Running is therapy for Missy. "It's my place to go and lose myself, whether I need to lose myself because it's been stressful and I need to let things go, or because I need to lose myself and just run. It's my place to feel better," she says.

Missy uses the principles of responsive endurance training by being aware that her body positively responds to physical activity, which alleviates her anxiety and depression symptoms. This self-awareness keeps her motivated because the benefits of exercise in her life are clear.

Relative Energy Deficiency in Sport

As consumers, there is immense pressure to buy into diet and exercise protocols that will help us lose weight quickly. Messages from social media influencers and those in the health and fitness industries often revolve around unrealistic standards of beauty that are tied to maintaining a thin physique. In the world of sport, there is often pressure for endurance athletes to achieve a lean "racing weight" to enhance speed and performance. In short: We live in a confusing world where we are bombarded with messages that do not always have a positive effect on our health.

This pressure to maintain a certain body composition puts additional stress on athletes because it can cause them to under-fuel, which puts them at risk for developing relative energy deficiency in sport (RED-S). Formerly known as female athlete triad, this syndrome was renamed to broaden the definition to include both men and women—anyone may be at risk of under-eating because they believe they need to restrict their food intake to support their training goals. According to the *British Journal of Sports Medicine*, RED-S refers to impaired physiological function that can affect metabolic rate, menstrual function, bone health, immunity, protein synthesis, and cardiovascular health.

Rebecca McConville, who, as mentioned in chapter 3, is a registered dietitian and expert on RED-S, says that RED-S is a mismatch of energy needs versus energy output. "The body is brilliant at preserving itself, so it will start slowing down other functions within the body like digestion, heart rate, estrogen production, and testosterone." When the body recognizes that there is not enough energy available (calories) for the activities demanded, the body will stop producing estrogen, which is needed to maintain bone density. So an athlete with RED-S puts herself at risk of osteopenia and osteoporosis. Rebecca says that the body prioritizes the training, and it slows down the other physiological functions, which are also required for good health.

In her book, *Finding Your Sweet Spot: How to Avoid RED-S (Relative Energy Deficit in Sport) by Optimizing Your Energy Balance*, some of the signs of RED-S Rebecca includes are loss of menstruation or irregular periods, lightheadedness or spotting in the eyes upon standing, decreased ability to maintain exertion, inability to sleep, disruptive sleep, stress reactions, stress fractures, increased length of time for recovery from injury, depressed mood, irritability, increased anxiety, inability to withstand training load, decreased endurance performance, and more.

Looking at the list, it's easy to see why RED-S can be difficult to diagnose. In fact, the *British Journal of Sports Medicine* says that less than 50 percent of clinicians and coaches are able to identify the components of RED-S. It is for this very reason that I have included a section on RED-S in this book. It is *critical* for you to understand that you *must* fuel your body properly for the activities you participate in.

Rebecca encourages athletes to find their sweet spots and optimize their nutritional and training plans to the activity as well as to the individual athlete. She cautions against strict dietary protocols and haphazard changes in exercise and nutrition. It's important to know why we make the changes and how they are affecting our health. If you begin seeing the warning signs of RED-S in yourself or your training partner, consult a sports dietitian who is well versed in this syndrome and in disordered eating.

This is precisely what responsive endurance training is all about: being observant and recognizing changes—both positive and negative—that take place as you fuel and train.

BE GOOD TO YOURSELF

Let's talk about stress. Exercise is one of the best tools for dealing with stress, anxiety, and depression. But sometimes we put so much pressure on ourselves to be perfect that exercise falls into the "have to" bucket instead of the "get to" bucket. If you are at a point where training feels like a chore, rather than something you look forward to—or you're feeling overwhelmed or have other signs of stress like chest pain, headaches, rapid heart rate, tension, or anger—it's time to take a step back. Cortisol, known as the stress hormone, wreaks havoc on our health when the body remains in fight-or-flight mode for extended periods of time.

If your training is excessive or isn't bringing you joy, it won't sufficiently decrease your stress.

Here are some additional tips for managing stress:

* Mindfulness and meditation can help reduce stress, and short bursts of time spent on focused breathing will restore a sense of calm. If you don't know where to start, search "mindfulness" in the app store. You'll find several apps that will lead you through breathing exercises that don't require a lot of time.
* Time with a friend or loved one can also provide stress relief. Combine this time with a mug of green tea or a walk outside, and you'll gain the benefits of multiple stress relievers merged into one.
* Snuggling with your dog, warm baths, massages, and hugs all release oxytocin, which has the opposite effect of cortisol on the system.

When we feel stressed, it can be hard to convince ourselves to take actions that will snap us out of the stressful situation, but sometimes help is as simple as a hug. In fact, Dr. Paul Zak, a world-renowned expert on oxytocin, says that receiving eight hugs a day releases the ideal level of oxytocin.

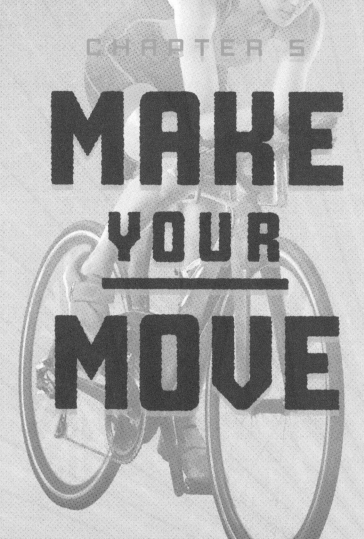

CHAPTER 5

MAKE
YOUR
MOVE

BY THE END OF THIS CHAPTER, you'll be ready to design and test your own RET strategy. First, we need to touch on a few more elements of a successful endurance strategy. Earlier, I mentioned that you'll need to make time for more than your primary endurance activity. You may become overwhelmed when you're trying to balance the demands of life with training, and now I'm sauntering in, asking you to add more. In the past, recreational athletes didn't put much thought into warm-ups, cool-downs, mobility, strength training, and rest. What coaches and runners now know is that these elements are all critical for longevity and injury-free participation in endurance sports. I firmly believe that mobility, strength, and rest are just as important as your swimming, biking, running, rowing, or climbing activities. Mobility and strength are not "extras" that you add in if you have the time. And, rest is not optional.

The topics discussed in this chapter are foundational. They are not like the bow on the top of the package, there for decoration. These are things that will make you stronger and more resilient as you pursue your passion.

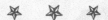

Mobility and Flexibility

Mobility is the ability of any joint to actively move through its full range of motion. The inability of a joint to move properly means that the body must contort into an unnatural position in order to complete the action. A cyclist lacking mobility in her back might not be able to ride in the aero position. A runner lacking mobility in his ankles might rotate his foot or hip in order to strike the ground comfortably.

People often use the terms *flexibility* and *mobility* interchangeably, but flexibility is the ability for the muscle to lengthen. When you see the Rockettes' high kicks or an ice-skater spin with her leg extended overhead, you are witnessing flexibility.

In truth, flexibility and mobility work together—it takes more to address movement issues than a little static stretching.

As you can imagine, repeated unnatural movement patterns can cause injuries. You might not notice that you lack range of motion in your hips while your training volume is low. However, as your training time increases, the weaknesses in your bio-mechanics will rear their ugly heads like Medusa's venomous snakes.

Let's cover a few of the basics:

BEFORE YOU START YOUR ACTIVITY, TAKE TIME TO WARM UP. It's common to see groups of runners standing around before a group run, stretching by pulling their legs behind them as they yank their heels to their butts. I often refer to this as old-school-gym-class stretching because it was common in the 1970s and '80s. It's ineffective and can cause injuries when you stretch a muscle that isn't warm.

Instead, start with a dynamic warm-up that elevates your heart rate and takes your muscles through their full range of motion, including the motions that are commonly used in your sport. In a dynamic warm-up, the body is in constant motion. Do not hold the stretch. Save the static stretching for after your workout when your muscles are warm.

INCORPORATE MOBILITY EXERCISES INTO YOUR DAY. You can incorporate mobility exercises into your warm-up or cool-down, or take breaks throughout your workday and do one or two exercises at the top of each hour. If you sit at a desk or spend a lot of time driving, you'll want to do exercises that will increase hip flexor mobility. Swimmers need mobility exercises for their shoulders and ankles. And nearly every runner I've ever met could use more ankle and hip mobility.

AFTER YOU EXERCISE, DO YOUR STATIC STRETCHING— AND INCLUDE SOME SOFT TISSUE WORK. The time to hold your stretches is when your muscles are warm. The National Academy of Sports Medicine recommends holding a stretch for 30 seconds to improve flexibility. I also recommend soft tissue work, such as foam rolling, to break up adhesions, increase blood flow, decrease soreness, and reduce muscle tension.

DON'T FORGET YOUR FEET! Your feet are your foundation, and if your foot doesn't move properly, it affects movement all the way up the kinetic chain. At a minimum, keep a tennis ball or lacrosse ball under your desk and spend a few minutes each day rolling the bottoms of your feet. My favorite resource for all things foot health is Dr. Emily Splichal, a podiatrist, human movement specialist, and global leader in barefoot science and rehabilitation. Her book, *Barefoot Strong*, is the go-to resource for improving foot health (see Resources on page 167).

Mobility is such an important topic, and I could fill multiple books with all you need to know. On my website, I include links to my favorite resources as well as some mobility playlists. Go to https://www.crushingmygoals.com for access to the latest updates.

Strength Training: Get Stronger to Get Faster

When I first started running, I was convinced I could finally be done with strength training. I was a runner with muscular legs. I didn't need to spend time with weights! As multiple injuries kept me sidelined, I sought answers: Why was I constantly getting injured? I completed my first coaching certification program with the single goal of getting the information I needed to finally stop the injury cycle.

I got what I came for. I left with knowledge that would help me avoid injury. But then I wondered why no one was talking about this stuff. Today, information on strength training for endurance athletes is extremely accessible via YouTube, Instagram, podcasts, books, and the web. But at the time it felt like a closely guarded secret.

All athletes need strength training. Strength training helps us maintain lean muscle mass, which is important for strength and power but is also a concern as we age. Because most endurance sports take place in one plane of motion (we are primarily moving forward, with little rotational or side-to-side movement), resistance training helps us strengthen muscles that are neglected. Strength training also boosts anaerobic capacity, helps you recruit the necessary muscle fibers to surge up a hill, gives you the power to push your speed at the end of a race, strengthens connective tissue, and makes your movement more efficient.

If you've ever wished that you had a fairy godmother who could wave her wand and grant you endurance superpowers, this is where the magic is!

Because most endurance runners don't love spending time in the gym, I prefer exercises that perform double duty by working multiple muscle groups at once. Total body strength is important, and a coach or trainer can help you assess your body for muscle imbalances and areas of weakness, allowing you to focus on the sections that will improve your performance the most.

All endurance athletes need a strong core, which encompasses the entire midsection—everything except the limbs—including the back, glute, and hip muscles, too. My tried-and-true exercises for core strength include planks, side planks, push-ups, tree choppers, and bird dogs.

Many lower body exercises also work the core. To work on glute, hip, and overall leg strength, I like exercises such as squats, single-leg dead lifts, single-leg squats, bridges, curtsy lunges, skaters, hip hikes, hamstring curls, clamshells, lunges, and lunges with a rotation.

The majority of the exercises listed above are bodyweight exercises, which are versatile because they can be completed at home, at work, or in a hotel (if you are someone who travels frequently). Your fitness progresses when you mix things up and continue to challenge yourself. If the base exercises become too easy, you can add bands, tubes, or weights to increase the difficulty. For best results, you want to work each muscle group two or three times per week, separated by at least a day for recovery.

If strength training is something you don't like to think about, consider working with a personal trainer who has knowledge of endurance sports. For additional variety, a class or session using suspension straps is also beneficial. TRX offers an app that will take you through a total-body workout—and I especially like this because suspension trap training is equally accessible for people of all abilities. If you have muscle weaknesses that affect your balance, or as you progress to a more challenging version of an exercise, the straps can help you maintain proper form.

A final option is to take a group fitness class that involves weights or a class with ballet-style movements, like barre. I'm also a huge fan of Orangetheory Fitness, but since most workouts tend to be hard days (according to the definitions we are using in this book), I recommend at least one rest day between sessions.

Rest to Be Your Best

Your body makes training adaptations while at rest, and if you don't take the time for proper recovery, you inhibit your body's ability to repair tissue, balance hormones, and restore energy. Without adequate rest, you also risk compromising your immune system, and you increase the likelihood of injury.

Rest is required.

In our society, it's a badge of honor to be in constant motion, to always be busy. However, downtime is beneficial for our health and athletic performance.

SLEEP Sleep feels good and restores the body. According to the National Sleep Foundation, adults need seven to nine hours of sleep a night, and athletes might require even more. If your sleep quality is lacking, attempt to go to bed at the same time each night. Sleep in a cool room, limit caffeine late in the day, and avoid blue light from televisions and other screens at least two hours before bed.

ALTERNATE HARD AND EASY EFFORTS In order for your body to have time to recover between training sessions, alternate hard days and easy days. Long runs and rides qualify as hard efforts, as do weight-training and high-intensity efforts. The day after a hard effort, include an easy or moderate intensity run or ride, full rest, or a restorative modality such as yoga.

PERIODS OF REDUCED TRAINING VOLUME A good plan also includes a "cutback" week, which takes place every three to five weeks and involves cutting training volume by 20 to 30 percent so the body gets additional rest.

It's also important to watch your body for signs of overtraining. If you experience insomnia or restless sleep, elevated resting heart rate, excessive fatigue, decreased performance, increased perceived exertion, moodiness, or increased injuries, your body could be telling you that it needs more rest.

If you notice a climb in your morning heart rate over a period of several weeks, you should incorporate additional rest days and stick with lower-intensity training until your heart rate returns to what is typical for you. Use a combination of the signs of over-training to assess your recovery. If you push through and ignore the warning signs, you will venture into dangerous territory that could have long-term effects on your health and ability to train.

Responsive endurance training requires that you listen to the signals your body sends. You will learn the difference between a day when you are seeking a reason to skip a workout and a day that your body is sending out an SOS. When your body is in distress, throw it a lifeline and incorporate additional rest.

Build Your Training Program

It is time to pull all this information together and build yourself a training program! As you develop your plan, you'll consider what we've discussed in previous sections. And you'll study your journal, keeping the principles of responsive endurance training in mind. Over time, you will discover how your body responds best. I've shared the big-picture things that can affect performance: nutrition, rest, mobility, strength, mind-set, and varied intensities of sport-specific training. Now it's time for you to fine-tune the details.

The Weekly Framework

Begin with the end in mind

When I create a training plan for a client, I start with the race date. If you're training without a race in mind, that's perfectly fine, but

WHY WE RACE
SHATTERING MARATHON RECORDS

For years, people speculated about whether it was possible for anyone to break the two-hour marathon barrier. Researchers from *Medicine & Science in Sports & Exercise* created a model that predicted a 10 percent likelihood of breaking two hours before May 2032, with only a 5 percent likelihood before 2024.

On October 12, 2019, Eliud Kipchoge, a 34-year-old Kenyan, made history, breaking the two-hour barrier. Although Kipchoge has the honor of being the first person to break two hours, the achievement is not considered an official world record because the event was planned and executed to allow circumstances that are not legal in normal competition. His time of 1:59:40 in the exhibition race is still a phenomenal feat, proving it's possible for the body to shatter beliefs about human potential.

The same weekend, Kenyan Brigid Kosgei beat Paula Radcliffe's world record time, which had stood for 16 years. The 25-year-old finished the Chicago Marathon with a time of 2:14:04, breaking the women's marathon world record by 81 seconds.

These achievements were not without controversy. Both athletes wore a prototype of the Nike Vaporfly NEXT%, a shoe that some say gives runners an unfair advantage. The Vaporfly is said to improve running economy by a minimum of 4 percent, and a *New York Times* analysis of 500,000 marathon and half marathon running times since 2014 confirms that "in a race between two marathoners of the same ability, a runner wearing Vaporflys would have a real advantage over a competitor not wearing them."

The International Association of Athletics Federations' (IAAF) rule 143.2 stipulates that shoes "must not be constructed so as to give athletes any unfair assistance or advantage." Though there is debate about what constitutes an unfair advantage, everyone does acknowledge the athleticism required to perform at the level of Kipchoge and Kosgei.

Dr. Mark Cucuzzella, author of *Run for Your Life*, says the shoe gives a technological advantage, and argues that there's a limit to what technology should be able to do. Because of the shoe's construction—a combination of foam and a carbon-fiber plate in the midsole—the shoe could be considered a spring, which is banned by the IAAF.

Time will tell how this new shoe technology plays out, but Dr. Cucuzzella says that the shoe isn't doing runners' feet any favors. He says the plate assists the big toe, supporting the stabilization and loading of the foot, which decommissions the muscles that should perform those functions. For someone who wants longevity as a runner, it would be healthier to run in a shoe that allows the foot to move as it is intended.

We live in exciting times with advancements that allow us to continue to push the limits of human performance. In 1954, Roger Bannister ran the first four-minute mile, proving the four-minute barrier could be broken. Now Eliud Kipchoge and Brigid Kosgei have given us new targets to aim for in the marathon.

it's important to know what you're working toward. Depending on your goal, you might want 12, 16, or 20 weeks to prepare. Once I know how long the training cycle will be, I draw a calendar grid on a sheet of paper, leaving enough rows for each week between the start of the plan and race day.

Block out rest days and long-workout days

Next, go through and block out at least one rest day a week, and note which day you want to complete your most time-intensive workout (your long run or long ride day).

Factor in high-intensity days

Once those pieces are in place, designate which days will be HIIT days. Keeping Dr. O'Keefe's guidelines in mind, schedule HIIT for one or two days per week—and remember that these are your hard days. If your workouts are short, these would be good days to also schedule your strength training. This allows you to keep the hard days hard and the easy days easy.

Add in the easy days

Now we have just the easy days left. Two of the easy days should be low to moderate intensity in your primary sport. If you are a runner, this will be an easy run day. If you cycle, this will be an easy ride day. The remaining easy day can be a form of cross-training, which I highly recommend. Cross-training gives you a means of working neglected muscle groups. It also provides a mental break, and it is a way to reconnect with friends who are not training for the same event as you. Sometimes training can feel intense or isolating, and you will be happier if you find ways to include friends and family in your training life. The bonus easy day is one way to incorporate a more playful workout into your plan.

Building

Now that we've discussed the weekly framework, let's talk about the duration of each workout. What is your starting point? What does your typical run, ride, or swim workout currently look like? And what is the longest distance you've gone over the past month? Start where you are, and then increase the distance by 10 to 20 percent per week.

The 10 percent rule comes from the "rule of toos": too much, too soon, too fast is a recipe for injury. However, this is a case where you should listen to your body. A 10 percent weekly increase in distance is conservative, but you also don't want to make huge leaps. Your muscles, tendons, and ligaments always need time to adapt to increases in distance. It's best if you factor a gradual increase in distance into your plan, rather than rushing to rack up big numbers quickly.

The next marks you'll make on the calendar relate to training phases. From race day, work back one week for a 5K or 10K, two weeks for a half marathon, and three weeks for a marathon. This is where your taper begins. The taper is where you cut back your mileage so that you get quality rest before race day.

Think in Phases

With the remaining weeks, start at the beginning of the plan and allocate four to six weeks for building endurance. Of course, you'll continue building endurance throughout the entire plan—but in this phase, you'll be especially conservative about making sure your body is prepared for more intense training. High-intensity work and speed work are limited in this phase. The goal is to safely build endurance while giving your muscles, tendons, and ligaments time to adapt to training.

The next block of training is a strength phase, and you'll spend about four weeks here. At the beginning of this phase, your high-intensity days will include small amounts of hill work with rest between each set. As you progress through the four-week period, the number of sets will increase—gradually. In this phase, you are increasing strength. Toward the end of this phase, you can also introduce plyometrics. Plyometric moves involve jumping or bounding. Some examples are box jumps, squat jumps, hill bounding, single-leg hops, and plyometric skaters. Again, start with a low number of repetitions and gradually build up the number over several weeks.

During the remaining weeks between the strength/hill phase and the taper, you will spend roughly four weeks working on speed. This is when your hard days are focused on longer portions at your projected race pace, and it's when you get in some serious speed work and interval training. Before you go hard-core into speed training, I recommend introducing fartlek runs (see page 30 for details). There are lots of ways to use fartleks, but one place is definitely as an introduction to speed work.

Arthur Lydiard, a New Zealand coach who heavily influenced American running during the running boom in the 1960s, had his runners incorporate hill bounding, which involves leaping strides up a 100- to 200-meter gentle hill. (See the reference link on page 176 for a demo video.) Lydiard also introduced periodized training, similar to the phases I'm recommending here. He believed that each system must be developed in order, and that the body was not prepared for anaerobic development (tempo runs and speed intervals) until after the hill/strength phase was complete. Most modern-day training programs began with Lydiard's theories as their foundation, but not all coaches today adhere to the same structure.

This is another example of where it pays to be conservative in your training, and it's also something you can track as you train year after year. Does your body respond best to sequential phases? Or do you progress better when you consistently mix distance, speed, and strength? No matter which approach you take, it's always best to make incremental changes.

A Few Additional Details

As you move through your plan using RET, you'll monitor how your body feels and adapt the plan accordingly. Consistency is one of the most important aspects of training, and the fastest way to become inconsistent is to overtrain or become injured.

If you find that you can't complete a long run once every seven days because your body requires more rest, consider adjusting your plan so that the long run or ride takes place every 10 or 14 days. There is nothing magic about the number seven, other than that it fits well on a calendar, so you know that each Monday or Saturday is the same type of workout from week to week. A long run every 10 days is better than a long run once every five weeks because you pushed beyond your body's capabilities.

Once you have the rough outline of your schedule, you'll also want to pencil in the cutback weeks. Space them out so that every three to five weeks you have reduced training volume. Keep in mind, though, that this is not a concrete rule. If you need a week with less intensity or volume sooner, do what your body tells you.

A lot goes into developing a training plan, but this is a rough framework to help you get started. If you decide to work with a coach, the same concepts apply, and you should communicate with your coach, keeping the responsive endurance training principles in mind. Your coach is only as good as the information you share. They are not inside your head, and they don't know what it feels like to live and train in your body. Work together so they can help you prepare with success—and longevity—in mind.

BE GOOD ᴛᴏ YOURSELF

If you are not feeling motivated to train, you might be able to blame dopamine. As one of the "feel good" neurotransmitters, dopamine makes us feel happy. It's tied to mood, sleep, memory, movement, and motivation. Dopamine levels spike in anticipation of activities that are rewarding, exciting, or pleasurable.

The day I ran my first half marathon, I was fatigued and I wanted to quit. I was excited about the session I had planned with a tattoo artist later that day, and anticipation of my new running tattoo (wings with a 13.1 in the middle) caused a dopamine spike that pushed me to keep going.

If you can learn to associate racing or training with something pleasurable or rewarding, it's possible for dopamine to give you that extra motivational boost.

Here are other ways you can get a surge of dopamine:

* Use your journal to record your training and racing achievements. When you flip through the journal, you'll begin to see training activities as being rewarding.
* Break a big goal (training for a marathon) into a series of mini goals, such as run a 5K, complete a 10K, and finish a half marathon. You'll stay motivated because you'll be rewarded with dopamine as you hit each smaller goal.
* Produce more dopamine naturally by eating foods that are sources of omega-3s, probiotics, vitamin D, and magnesium, to name a few.

If all else fails, and you need to pump up your motivation or mood, find something to laugh about. A date night at the comedy club or a few minutes on the phone with a friend who always tickles your funny bone should do the trick.

CHAPTER 6

THE

MENTAL GAME

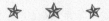

WE ARE ONLY now beginning to understand the ways that thoughts affect human behavior and performance. The words we repeat to ourselves dictate our beliefs, and therefore our actions. If we believe we are destined to fail, that belief influences our resilience. Rather than working through a tough situation, we are more likely to give up. Likewise, if we believe that it's possible to remain mentally sharp and live an active lifestyle into our 90s, we are more likely to choose lifestyle habits that make that vision become a reality.

The words we tell ourselves matter. That internal dialogue that runs in the background as you go about your day can set you up for success or contribute to your struggles. Once you become aware of how powerful your thoughts are, you can take more control of your mental habits.

In this chapter, we'll talk about how to manage your mind, using it to protect your well-being and boost your performance. We will look at how optimism and visualization affect athletic performance, how to cultivate mental toughness, and how you can use your journal to do mental work that leaves you feeling strong and capable. We'll also look at strategies for incorporating the lessons from this book into your life, and end with some ideas to help you relax so you can put your body in situations that rejuvenate and feed your soul.

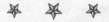

The Mind and Performance

Successful athletes use optimism, positive self-talk, and visualization to gain a competitive edge. But it's more than a performance-enhancing strategy to help you dominate during your next half marathon. This is one of my favorite topics because I believe it's possible for anyone to influence the trajectory of their life by learning to harness the power of their mind. This is more than New Age thinking. There's lots of scientific and empirical evidence that this stuff works.

Optimism

When you are in a place of gratitude, optimism, and positivity, you are sending your body the signals it needs to thrive. I interviewed Olympic marathoner Deena Kastor for my podcast, and she shared how her life was transformed as she learned to cultivate optimism. Shortly after graduating from college, she went to work with coach Joe Vigil. "He talked about an athlete's lifestyle and how it's not just about showing up for practice for two hours in the day. It's how you live your entire day that adds up to either supporting or diminishing your efforts as an athlete," she said. "It was so eye-opening to me, and it made me excited to finally tap in and see what my potential was."

Deena explained that achievements are determined by more than the traits we are born with. "After talking to Coach Vigil, I immediately got into this growth mind-set, just wanting to learn and expand and absorb everything he taught." She was prepared to take on the challenge of training with Coach Vigil and says she realized from the first week that enthusiasm and excitement played a huge role in how she adapted at altitude.

She quickly realized that the voice in her head that said, "I'm so tired" or "I hate this hill" had her defeated before she even got to the workout or before she approached the incline to the hill. But if she flipped the script and said, "This hill will make me stronger. Each time I climb this, I'm getting stronger," the change in mind-set dramatically changed the outcome of that little moment. This led her to realize that if she could continue to change little moments back-to-back-to-back, that would significantly change the experience. From there, it became a game to her.

By paying closer attention to everything happening around her, Deena found opportunities to adjust her thoughts in order to become her own advocate and a cheerleader, rather than a critic. "We are our best critics, but to be our best cheerleaders and our best advocates is the most important thing," she said. "We have control over that. Our minds are malleable, and our brains are just patterns of thought processes. If we can change those patterns to be more positive, more uplifting, and more empowering, we are getting the best out of our physical bodies to reach our potential."

Deena initially made the mind-set changes because she wanted to be a faster, stronger, more enduring runner, but she noticed her new mind-set had a profound effect on her daily life as well. "It was making my days more beautiful and compassionate and understanding," she said. "Then I added gratitude lists to the mix, and my world exploded." She said that gratitude made her take notice of the world around her. "We tend to take in a lot of the negativity that happens around us, but if we pause for a second to appreciate all the good and beauty and opportunity that's happening simultaneously, then the negativity tends to recede into the background, and it feels like you're living a pretty abundant life."

Deena is the perfect example of an athlete who uses the principles of responsive endurance training to get the most out of herself. In her memoir, *Let Your Mind Run: A Memoir of Thinking My Way to Victory*, Deena shares how the practice of cultivating optimism changed her life and her career.

Visualization

Your brain can't tell the difference between reality and visualization. Great runners spend hours visualizing every aspect of the racecourse: the crowds, the hills, their own relaxed running form, and the way they surge past competitors in the race to the finish. Mental rehearsal allows us to prepare for our athletic goals.

If you experience prerace anxiety, try mentally rehearsing how you'll navigate the race before it begins. Imagine what could transpire and mentally work your way through these possible events until you have an action plan for dealing with every tricky situation you could encounter.

Most importantly, visualize success. This is more than theoretical. There are a number of studies (see the references for chapter 6 on page 177) that demonstrate that mental rehearsal helps reduce strength loss in injured athletes who need to rehabilitate after ACL surgery. Other studies have shown that simply observing someone exercise can result in physiological responses, such as increased heart rate, respiration, and blood pressure. Some experts believe that mental practice is as effective as physical practice and could be used alongside physical practice to reduce overtraining and overuse injuries. It might be hard to believe that mental rehearsal creates neural pathways in your brain, but it's true. Consistent mental rehearsal has the potential to cut physical training time in half, according to some studies.

Mental rehearsal can help certain behaviors become habit, and helps you become familiar with race day routines. Knowing that you've experienced certain aspects of the race—even if it's only been through visualization—can calm your nerves and help you focus when it counts. I mentally rehearse triathlon transitions, picturing how I will set up my transition area. I imagine running up the beach from the swim, ripping my swim cap off, sitting on a towel next to my bike, slipping on my socks, then shoes, placing my sunglasses on my face, and snapping my helmet into place as I stand to pull my bike off the rack. I go through this mental routine for weeks before triathlon season begins. Because of this mental rehearsal, my transitions are quick and on task.

What to Do with Discomfort

The best performance-enhancing tool we have is the power of our own mind. Many athletes repeat power phrases, words of affirmation, or mantras to themselves. Multiple studies show that self-talk reduces the rate of perceived exertion, which means you can literally talk yourself out of being exhausted—and ultimately increase your endurance. Anything that affects the perception of effort will improve endurance performance. This means that listening to music or a motivational podcast, reciting Bible verses, or repeating mantras can boost performance if the tactic is something that helps you avoid thinking about how hard you're working. It's all individual, and what helps one athlete might not work for another. Again, you'll want to try several approaches to see what helps you most.

When thinking about dealing with discomfort while training and racing, it's important to know the difference between *needing* to stop because you are dehydrated or injured and *wanting* to stop because you're tired or no longer want to deal with the discomfort. To be clear: Never continue the activity in a situation that could negatively affect your life or health. That may seem obvious, but in our no-pain-no-gain society, there is pressure to persevere.

When I talk about mental toughness, I'm talking about that juncture in every endurance event when you begin to battle your own mind. Mental toughness can be learned, as can strategies for redirecting your attention when you feel like giving up.

When you hit your threshold and need to take your mind off the pain, start with a form check. If you're running, think about your posture: Are you running tall with your chin in a neutral position? Are your feet landing under your center of mass? Are your arms relaxed? What about your shoulders? Are they tense and tucked under your ears or are they loose?

Next, focus on breathing. Take some deep breaths in, bringing air deep into your abdomen, and exhale slowly. Try counting steps as you fill your body with oxygen and imagine energy being delivered to every muscle, from your head to your toes.

Check your nutrition. Do you need fuel? When was the last time you had something to drink? There is some evidence that swishing a drink containing a sugar solution and spitting it out can boost endurance and trick the brain into thinking more energy is on the way. (This is especially effective if you're experiencing GI distress and can't keep liquids down.)

After you've checked in with yourself physically, it's time to turn to mental tactics. Mantras can be an incredibly effective way to boost your endurance and distract you from your discomfort. Come up with a power phrase or a few phrases to repeat to yourself when times get tough. You can repeat things like:

I am strong.

I love hills.

Hills make me stronger.

I have energy.

There is some research that shows that mantras can be more effective when they are repeated in the second person (*You are strong*), so like everything with responsive endurance training, test it and see which method works best for you.

If you are racing and you decide it's not your day, there's no harm in taking it easy. In the Boston Marathon edition of my podcast, my friend Bill Williams shared the story of his experience at the Fargo Marathon. He had a race where nothing was going right, so he decided to make the best of it and just have fun. He talks about interacting with the crowd, stopping in on a birthday party, taking a few hops across a trampoline, and generally living in the moment.

I think that is the most important lesson of all. YOU decide how your day is going to go. Responsive endurance training is about accepting where you are in the moment and doing what is best for YOU. We don't have to try to get a personal record each time we race. Sometimes the fun is in finding a way to persevere, to release our preconceived expectations, and to have fun—especially when the day isn't going as planned.

WHY WE RACE
RAISING HEALTHY YOUNG ATHLETES

There is tremendous pressure for kids to start sports—and begin specializing in one—at a young age. The National Athletic Trainers' Association (NATA) released a statement aimed at reducing the risk of injury due to sports specialization at an early age. Their recommendations included kids participating in a variety of sports to encourage development of athletic skills, playing on only one team at a time, limiting weekly sports participation to no more hours than their age, and including two full rest days per week.

Kids can learn valuable life lessons through their participation in sports, and they will have a stronger athletic future if the focus is on becoming a well-rounded athlete. Although sports can help children develop a strong work ethic, it's best to take the focus off competition and, instead, help the young athlete learn the value of teamwork, how to set goals, what it means to be a good teammate, how to learn from losses and disappointment, how to manage stress, and how to have compassion for themselves and others.

No matter which sports kids participate in, we need to talk to them about more than the game or the specific event. Conversations should center on helping them learn skills that will affect lifelong success. Developing a lifestyle and work ethic that support our goals plays a bigger role in success than natural talent.

When I asked Deena Kastor what she would tell her younger self, she told me that as a younger athlete, she lined up at the starting line every weekend just thinking, "I hope my talent holds today. I hope it holds out for one more race." She said she knew people praised her talent and meant it as a compliment, but it took many years before she realized she was the driving force—and that her success was due to more than talent. Because of that experience, she would tell her younger self: *Don't listen to anyone who says you're talented. You've worked hard for the privilege of this first-place finish, and you have to continue working hard. It happens in practice.*

You Need to Chill

The type A behaviors that make you successful in life and at work also give you a competitive edge in sports. While you need your fire and drive, you also need to balance that energy in order to reach your full potential. The rest and recovery methods discussed earlier cover the physical breaks that are specific to training. This section is an invitation to pause for some soothing inner work. I want to encourage you to sit down every week to reflect on your athletic pursuits and on life in general.

When I don't take time to reflect or slow down and recharge, I notice that my emotions are flat. I'm not excited about my work or my training, and the parts of my personality that make me feel alive aren't as evident. I personally need time to walk with my dogs (while listening to a podcast to fill my brain with positivity) and time to think about life, whether that involves problem-solving as I walk, or reflecting in my journal.

Using Your Journal

The missing piece in most training plans is a journaling component. I'm not talking about the old "dear diary" of your youth. And I'm not talking about simply logging your activity and nutrition. People who take the time to write and reflect each day are more likely to develop new habits and keep them long-term. That is why later in this book there is a section on how to create your own training journal (page 119).

When you record how you felt during your workout, or life challenges that come to mind, you can see patterns emerge. This can heighten your awareness of both positive and negative emotions that affect you as an athlete and a person who wishes to grow in general.

Journaling is a powerful tool that can help you enhance your life. Don't we all want to be dreamers, believers, and solution seekers? Whether you are an athlete who wants to achieve a new personal best, an employee going for a promotion, a forty-something just trying to get a handle on her food choices, or a mother with a chronic illness, you can use journaling to connect the dots between thoughts and behaviors—and do the work that supports your success.

Growth is messy. It's not perfect. And you don't have to think or feel the same way tomorrow that you feel today. The important thing is that you get something in the journal so that you have something to go back to. It's hard to start with a blank page, so write something today. Then when you start tomorrow, you're no longer staring at a blank page, and you have something to build on.

Some questions to help you get started:

* How do I feel right now mentally and physically?
* How do I feel about my training?
* Are there any negative thought patterns dragging me down?
* What do I wake up excited about each morning?
* Do I regard myself with compassion?
* What's propelling me forward?
* What have I done lately to recharge my batteries?
* What are the top 10 things I'm grateful for right now?
* What have I done lately just for fun?

Cultivating Inner Strength through Mind-and-Body Work

You might think that mindfulness and meditation practices are for flower children of the 1970s, but mindfulness practices have gone mainstream as more people recognize the benefits of an integrated approach to wellness. Because we finally have fancy technology that can be used to measure brain activity, enthusiasm for mind-and-body approaches to health is at a high point. There's now science to back what yogis and mindfulness practitioners have known all along. Mind-and-body practices cultivate inner strength and also enhance overall health.

Earlier, I mentioned that you should reserve at least one day a week as a rejuvenation day. While you could spend that day lounging in PJs and binge-watching Netflix, restorative practices that help you take a physical and mental break or connect with nature will do more for your mind and body. These restful activities are a great way to involve a friend or family member in your training. You can try some new classes, get outside, or download an app and experience something new together.

Qigong and Tai Chi

Restorative practices such as qigong and tai chi have ancient roots and are recognized as meditative movements that nourish the soul and keep us out of fight-or-flight mode. Both disciplines are typically categorized as meditative movement. The website for the National Qigong Association describes qigong as a "mind-body-spirit practice that improves one's mental and physical health by integrating posture, movement, breathing technique, self-massage, sound, and focused intent." Tai chi also involves slow, flowing movements that incorporate meditation and breath work.

Time in Nature

If you've ever felt at peace and centered after standing barefoot on the beach or looking out at the ocean, you already know that time in nature is good for you. Forest bathing, which is sometimes called ecotherapy, refers to spending time in nature. You do not need to hike into a famous national park or seclude yourself deep in the woods to benefit from forest bathing. You can achieve great benefits from spending just two hours weekly in a natural environment close to you. This could mean taking your dog for a walk through a neighborhood with lots of trees, having a picnic lunch in the park, or watching birds from a swing in your backyard. There are no rules for forest bathing, only that you spend time connecting with nature through your senses. For best results, put your phone away, move slowly, and drink in the sights, sounds, smells, and colors of the season.

Restorative Yoga

Restorative yoga is a calming style of yoga that involves passive holds and the use of props to enhance relaxation. It does not involve active stretching or holding the challenging poses you experience in other forms of yoga. Don't expect to break a sweat in a restorative yoga session; it should leave you feeling relaxed and refreshed.

Meditation

There are so many types of meditation, no one can agree on the number. What is important to know about meditation is that you don't need to overcomplicate it, and you can choose the style that you find most comfortable. To get started, you can use an app like Headspace, or you can sit quietly with your eyes closed for as little as one minute. Don't worry about rules or how long you're able to clear your mind. It's common to find meditation challenging, so jump in and build the duration by a minute or two with each session. One minute a day will provide more health benefits than avoiding meditation altogether, so don't be intimidated.

All these mind-and-body practices, which are backed by science, provide benefits such as increased focus, reduced stress, enhanced immune function, improved sleep quality, and a reduction in anxiety and depression. Other benefits include reduced risks of type 2 diabetes, cardiovascular disease, premature death, preterm birth, and high blood pressure. Studies on forest bathing also noted a reduction in the level of salivary cortisol, which is a marker of stress.

BE GOOD ᴛᴏ YOURSELF

One of my favorite interviews was when I talked with Nick Symmonds for my podcast. Nick is a two-time Olympian who has focused on the 800 meter for the majority of his career. Recently retired from professional running, he is also the cofounder and CEO of Run Gum. I ended the interview, as I do on every podcast, by asking him what traits he believed all champions possess. "To be a champion in anything," he said, "it takes perseverance. To get to the top, to be successful, curveballs and obstacles will be thrown your way, and you have to persevere. That's number one by a long shot."

Then, his thoughts turned to gratitude. "There's no point in doing any of this," he said, "if you're not going to look back and be grateful." He explained that he knows Olympic gold medalists who look back on their careers with nothing but frustration and disappointment because they never got the world record. And he knows world record holders who look back on their careers with disappointment and sadness because they never won an Olympic gold. "Stop and appreciate how cool that is, how hard you worked, and thank yourself for putting that hard work in," Nick said.

I have to agree. What is the point in doing all the things we do if we can't take some time to reflect and be grateful? Make a list of some of your accomplishments in life and sport. Think of this as your highlight reel. The next time you are down or feeling frustrated because you had a rough workout, pull out your highlight reel. Relive the moments, and take the time to be grateful for all the good in your life.

Gratitude can change your brain, make you more optimistic, reduce anxiety, improve your sleep, and even enhance your fitness. I think it's pretty cool that something that makes us feel good about ourselves is backed by science, too.

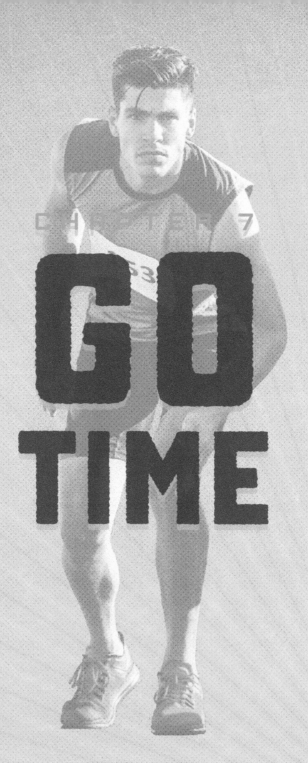

CHAPTER 7

GO TIME

HOW DO YOU KNOW if you're ready to race? I find that without a goal on the calendar—without a deadline—most people will never be ready because they will continue to procrastinate. Having a race in mind when you start training forces you to do the work. If you do the work and stick with your plan, you will be prepared on race day.

I am constantly reminding friends that endurance sports should be about having fun. Some people put off competition because they don't want to be the last one across the finish line, or the person who has to stop and walk during a marathon. I want you to put fear aside; stop worrying about what other people think. I assure you there are people of all fitness levels and ability levels on the racecourse, and everyone will be rooting for you. We are one big endurance family, and if you are out there with us, doing what we love, you are part of the family, too.

Ready to Race?

Whether you've participated in endurance sports your entire life or you picked up this book because you had a specific training goal in mind, you might be curious about endurance sports you haven't yet tried. I started out working with a trainer to develop strength and found myself running. When I became an injured runner, I turned to swimming. And from there, I developed an interest in triathlon. You never know when you'll be inspired to try something new.

Running

With running, you have several distances to choose from. In addition to the 5K, 10K, half marathon, and marathon, there's trail running and ultrarunning. Most people start with a 5K, which is 3.1 miles, and work their way up in distance from there. As we talked about earlier in the book, your body needs time to adapt, so increase your distance slowly.

You will probably want to use some combination of running and walking as you transition from walker to runner. Even after you've been running for years, there's no shame in walking. I recommend using a combination of running and walking for anyone coming back from illness or injury, as well as for anyone who wants to extend their mileage while reducing their risk of injury. Jeff Galloway popularized the run-walk-run method, and you can learn more about run-walk strategies for runners of all levels on his website.

In larger cities, you can easily find one or more 5K races to compete in every weekend. In addition to local half marathons and marathons, you might discover you enjoy the opportunity to see the world, exploring new cities 13.1 miles at a time. Whether you run for fun, to push your limits, or for the glory of standing on the podium, running can change your life.

Walking and Race Walking

Walking can be an incredible form of exercise—as well as a challenging competitive event that is included in the Olympics and Senior Games. Ten thousand years ago, our ancestors spent 10 to 14 hours a day moving, hunting, and gathering, and now we spend an average of 10 hours a day sitting. We were born to move. Our sedentary lifestyles have put us at greater risk for heart disease, type 2 diabetes, dementia, cancer, obesity, and more. Nearly everyone can walk, and you can get in your 30 minutes a day (without breaking a sweat!) during your lunch break at work.

If you opt for race walking or competitive race walking, there are a few form differences you must maintain. According to USA Track and Field, one foot must be in contact with the ground at all times, and the leading leg must remain straightened until the leg passes under the body. Just because *walking* is part of the name, don't think race walking is a leisurely stroll in the park. Top race walkers achieve paces of seven to eight miles per hour. You can look for race walking events in your area, or you can walk in any running event. If you choose to walk a half marathon or marathon, check the rules to see how long the course will remain open. Most races these days are walker-friendly, but if you're going to pay to compete, you want to be sure the same services available to runners will be there for you when you cross the finish line.

Swimming

Swimming is not just for high school and college kids. According to the US Masters Swimming (USMS) website, there are more than 500 local or regional competitions for adult swimmers in the United States each year, but fewer than half of USMS members compete in meets or open-water events. Triathletes often join masters swim programs because it's a good way to improve technique. Don't let the word *masters* scare you. Most sports have a masters designation, but it doesn't refer to skill. Rather, it refers to age, and a masters swimmer is anyone over 18.

When people tell me they want to do a triathlon, the sentence often ends with "but I don't know how to swim." I took swimming lessons as a kid, but I never got good enough to swim for exercise, until the year I hurt my hip while I was training for a marathon. A friend suggested that I join her in the pool for some cross-training, but before I could do that, I needed to become a stronger swimmer. We gathered a group of five people who met Coach Terry at the gym twice a week, and together we improved our swimming skills. Some of the group went on to compete in adult swim meets, and we all completed our first sprint triathlon together.

If you are new to swimming, it helps to find a coach or to join the masters swim program at a local gym. Your skills will improve more quickly if you have someone who can help you with technique.

Cycling

Cycling is a sport that is accessible to almost anyone, and the only gear you need is a bike, a helmet, and some sunglasses. For recreational riding, you can google "bike trails near me" to find a safe and scenic place to ride. To make a vacation of it, you can search for longer routes that take you across multiple states, like the 1,853-mile Pacific Coast Route or the 2,493-mile Great Divide Trail. Many trails are a mix of paved roads, gravel, and limestone, so you will want to choose a bike that can handle these surfaces. (You could take your road bike on a gravel ride, but you'll spend a lot of time changing flats, and the ride won't be as smooth.)

Cyclists can search online or visit a bike shop to find out about weekly group rides. These rides are usually categorized by average miles per hour, and the description should indicate whether the ride is a "no drop" ride, which means that no one is left behind, regardless of speed. Most communities have several larger organized rides each season, often to benefit a charity. These rides are "supported" rides, which means volunteers will be available to help change flats, assist with medical needs, and provide snacks on the course.

When you first start riding, it's a good idea to join a local bike club, so you can learn how to ride safely on the road and in groups. Always wear a helmet and protective eye covering. According to the American Association of Neurological Surgeons, concussions from cycling-related accidents outnumber concussions from football, softball, and baseball combined. If you ever crack your helmet, make sure you replace the helmet before your next ride.

Triathlon

Triathlon is made up of three events: swimming, biking, and running, completed in that order. Most people start with the sprint distance, which varies by venue but is usually a 500- to 750-meter swim, 10- to 15-mile bike ride, and 3.1-mile run. Longer races include the Ironman—which is a brand name that has become synonymous with the distances—and the half Ironman. The full Ironman distance is a 2.4-mile swim, 112-mile bike ride, and 26.2-mile run.

The biggest challenge when training for a triathlon is balancing the swim, bike, and run training. Because there are three disciplines and a lot of gear to juggle, triathlon can be the most intimidating endurance sport for beginners. You'll find a welcoming community that is willing to help you learn and advance your skills. While some triathletes go all out, spending thousands of dollars on fancy bikes, it's possible to start your triathlon journey with the bike you already have.

I did a series of podcasts covering common triathlon questions and topics, and you can find all my resources here: https://www .crushingmygoals.com/triathlon-resources.

WHY WE RACE
SEASONS OF LIFE AS AN ATHLETE

Some of my best running and triathlon memories are not about specific workouts, the time spent training, or even the events themselves. Instead, I smile when I think about the trips, the laughter, the silly photos, and the quiet early morning conversations between friends. I've loved having races to train for, goals to chase, and distances to conquer, but in the end the one thing that really stands out is the people who have touched my life as we pursued our goals.

The people you train with become like family, so love them while you can. We all go through different seasons of life, and your training partners and their availability will change, just as your own life ebbs and flows. Take the pressure off and shed the expectations. You don't need to be anyone other than who you are today, so appreciate your now.

It's easy to get caught up in the competitive spirit of the people around you or to see things online that cause you to believe that there's only one way to be an athlete. But the truth is, the way you look at endurance sports will change over the course of your life. When my kids were little, running was my lifeline. It brought me my own group of friends, a reason to get out of the house alone, and time to clear my mind and de-stress. During this time, I was learning to be a runner, and the time I spent training was largely social.

As my kids got older, it was easier to get out of the house. With more time to train, I turned my focus to triathlon. I made new friends, found new challenges, and loved that there was always something new to learn. Just as I found my groove, I was diagnosed with breast cancer.

While I recovered from my bilateral mastectomy, I gathered friends for long walks. When it was time for chemotherapy, I set a goal of running a 5K for each round of chemo. At the end of treatment, my friends joined me in a celebratory half marathon. Running took on a different meaning for me in this time of my life. It was a distraction and a way of reminding myself that I was strong.

Once my hair grew back, and there were no obvious signs of the trauma I'd endured, I was embarrassed to race again. If I had ever had any speed in my past, it was gone. And I now had joint, foot, and ankle pain that made running challenging. I finally realized I was letting my fears dictate what I did for fun. I was so worried that people might make fun of me that I stopped racing and training in groups. It took me longer than I'd like to admit to take my own advice and get past this.

In the summer of 2019, I decided it was time to embrace the season of life I am in. That meant doing what I could, competing for myself, and not being concerned about other people's opinions. Once I was confident that I could easily swim the 500-meter distance for the swim portion (because safety is important in water sports!), I signed up for two sprint triathlons. I did them for fun—and I had the absolute best time without having any expectations or pressure.

When you find that you are being tough on yourself because you're not hitting the times you did in the past or you're feeling more distracted than usual, give yourself some grace. Our endurance pursuits look different in different seasons of life. Rather than fight ourselves, sometimes it's best to be kind to ourselves. Honor your body and everything taking place, and appreciate who you are in this moment.

Race Week Training

In the days leading up to your race, you'll reduce your training volume so your body and mind can be in peak form for race day. Many athletes find the taper to be somewhat nerve-racking because they've become accustomed to high-volume training. They now have more time on their hands and are lacking an outlet for their energy. They might feel out of sorts because they are missing out on their daily endorphin hit. With training volume reduced, many athletes worry about losing fitness as they cut back on training to rest up.

Athletes whose training was hit-and-miss may suddenly find their motivation and have a strong desire to train hard in an attempt to make up for lost time. It's important to note that you will not make any fitness gains during race week that will help you in the short-term. This isn't like a test you can cram for; any intense, high-volume training done this week will only deplete your energy.

It's common to feel like something is "off" during the taper. Athletes often refer to this stage as having the "taper crazies" because it can feel unsettling to cut back on volume after months of focusing daily on getting each workout in. If you've adopted the responsive endurance training philosophy, you'll have some additional tools to calm your nerves.

Remember that recovery is critical if you want to perform your best on race day. Since you treated rejuvenation as a foundational rather than an optional piece of your plan, things like restorative yoga, time in nature, meditation, and taking time to play have been part of your training all along. Now you'll place more emphasis on restorative practices and less emphasis on physically demanding activities.

Flip through your journal this week and reflect on all the hard work that's gotten you this far. You'll see how you persevered. You'll be reminded of the tough workouts. You'll remember how you conquered hills and endured stormy weather. The pages of your journal should put your mind at ease. The experiences you documented made you the athlete you are today, the one who is prepared to stand on the start line.

Race Week Nutrition

Increase your carb intake slightly this week so that your muscles are replenished with glycogen. This doesn't mean it's time to eat all the ice cream, candy, and chips that cross your path. Continue to focus on quality, nutrient-dense carbohydrates. There will be plenty of time for a celebratory meal after the race.

Hydration should be a focus every day of your life, but during race week, it's especially important. Your water bottle should be your best friend this week, and you should have the goal of having pale and odor-free urine at the end of each day. You don't want to get to race day dehydrated, because drinking a ton of water right before you race will only lead to extra stops at the racecourse porta potties.

Attending a pasta party to carb-load with friends is a time-honored tradition among athletes. It's a great social outlet, and you get to talk about your race with others who are feeling the same excitement and jitters as you. It's best if your carb-loading takes place two days before the race, rather than the night before. This allows your body to store the fuel, and you won't have a bunch of heavy food sitting in your gut on race morning.

The Day before Your Race

You'll probably stop at the race expo to get your race bib, which you'll wear on your clothing during the race so that officials can identify you. If you've traveled for the race, it can be exciting to spend your day sightseeing after you've checked out the vendors at the expo. Remember that you have lots of distance to cover in the morning, and you don't want tired legs and feet. Pace yourself, wear comfortable shoes, and try to get to bed early.

That evening, consume easily digestible, low-fiber carbs that you've tested in training. If you've traveled to a race, it can be tempting to check out a new restaurant and consume exotic dishes you can't get at home. Stick with familiar foods that you know your digestive system can handle. Your body will thank you on race day when it's not diverting energy to the digestive system because the tuna casserole didn't agree with you.

Another note about your race bib: Sometimes you'll hear about athletes offering to give their race bib to a friend when they get injured or have a family event pop up on race day. Never take a bib without going through the transfer protocol the race director has in place. Competing as another athlete affects the race results. If you place while running as your friend and you aren't in that age or gender grouping, you've just cheated someone else out of their rightful slot. There's also a safety factor: The race bib is tied to the waiver the original bib owner signed when they registered, which means it's also associated with that person's emergency contact information. While serious accidents and injuries are rare, the officials need the emergency documentation for the person racing.

If you're new to racing, you'll want to avoid this newbie mistake: You'll receive an awesome shirt at the expo, and you'll be jazzed about wearing it. Call it a superstition, but it's tradition to wear the shirt after the race, not before. There's no harm in wearing the shirt, but as a newbie, it feels so much better to have it on while you're basking in your first postrace glow.

Race Day

When race morning finally arrives, you'll be running on adrenaline. Most athletes pack up their race gear the night before and wake up with their clothing all laid out. You will have enough nervous-excited energy without scrambling to find your shoes, sunglasses, visor, or watch.

Race Day Fueling

Some athletes have elaborate nutrition routines that involve waking up three to four hours before the race to begin fueling. I like to keep it simple by consuming a banana with peanut butter before heading out the door. I sip on an electrolyte drink, such as Nuun, until about five minutes before the race starts. Of course, this also means that I need to stand in line to visit the extremely posh facilities for one last potty break.

Stick with what's worked for you in training. This is why you test fuels throughout the training process—nutrition is individual, and you need to know how your nutrition affects your body: which foods leave you feeling energized and which foods move through your body too quickly. For a longer race, you'll want to consume calories throughout.

Some nutritionists recommend carrying your own drink with an electrolyte solution and consuming real food (a small sandwich, some applesauce, or diced potatoes) as you race. Others suggest using chews and gels and the drinks served on the course. Again, this is individual, and you'll need to test your nutrition in training. Most specialty running and cycling shops have an entire wall devoted to fueling products, so experiment in training and see what works best for you.

You've done the training, and you've taken care of the tiny details. Now it's time to toe the line!

You set a goal months ago, and you worked toward it consistently. Race day is a celebration of your accomplishments. You set out to be happy, healthy, and strong on race day, and now that it's here—enjoy the moment.

Onward

As I'm sure you've realized, there is no one best way to train. The best way is whichever way works for you, and the only way you'll know is to become adept at interpreting the messages your body sends you. Throughout the book, I have shown you where to look and taught you how to listen. We have covered a lot of ground: heart rate training, nutrition strategies, mobility and strength, rest and relaxation, and mind-set and habit creation. Along the way, I've encouraged you to record your findings and check in with yourself by creating a training journal.

By tracking what you try, how you feel, and how you perform, you'll uncover the best way to train for YOU. That best way will change as your goals and priorities shift, and I encourage you to treat yourself with compassion and accept what your body is capable of on each day and in each stage of life.

Responsive endurance training can lead to many years of successful fitness, competition, and vitality. Keep it up, keep listening to your body, and have fun. Your journey begins now.

BE GOOD TO YOURSELF

Sometimes endurance endeavors fill the empty space that's present in our souls when we feel we are lacking purpose. Although running and cycling provide mental health benefits and can boost your mood, it's not likely that running itself will bring long-term happiness or meaning to your life. Throughout training, you'll learn things about yourself that you didn't expect, and you'll encounter people who change your perspective or touch your life in a meaningful way. Running absolutely brings people and experiences into our lives that can help us feel whole, but have you ever found yourself wondering if there's more to life?

As you've searched for meaning and purpose in your own life, what have you noticed that makes you feel content? When you think about times when you are your most authentic self, who are you with, and what are you doing? What activities fill your life with meaning and purpose?

Take some time to contemplate what's most important to you. Create a list of the top 10 people, places, and activities that give you joy. How can you make room for more of these things in your life?

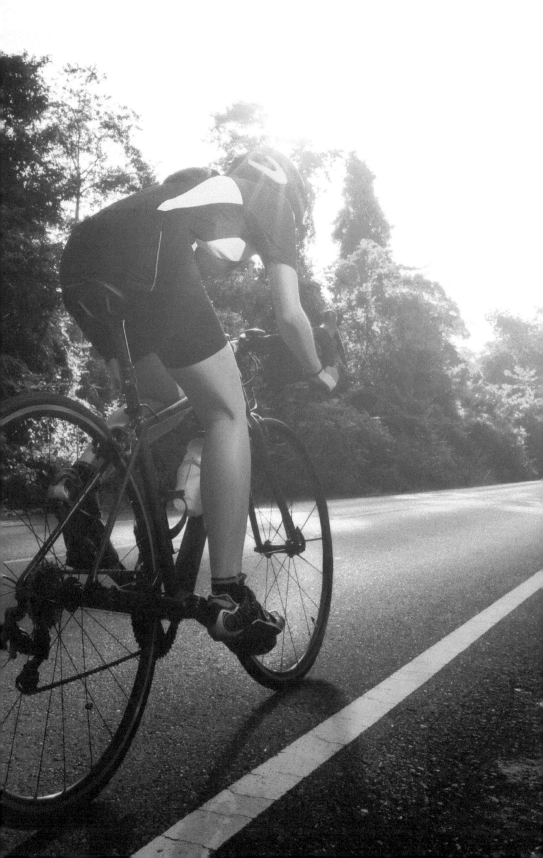

TRAINING JOURNAL
EXAMPLE

Your training journal doesn't need to be fancy. It can be a leather-bound notebook, a three-ring binder with loose-leaf paper, a spiral notebook—or any other method of tracking and recording that you dream up. I love using colorful fine-tipped markers and a few stickers from the craft store, but use whatever works for you. Play around with the type of information you want to track from day to day and week to week. You can use the ideas presented earlier in the book as well as the suggestions below to customize your journal so it's a valuable training tool.

Things you might want to track:

Date

Training method

Distance

Pace

Heart rate during training

Morning heart rate

Completion time

Route

Time of day

Meals and snacks

Daily hydration tracking

How I felt before training

How I felt during training

How I felt after training

What I did well

Areas that need more work

Mood

Mantras

Race day visualization exercises

Recovery methods

Gratitude practice ....

....

What gives me joy ....

....

What I'm looking forward to ....

....

Did I make time for my strength, mobility, and mindfulness
sessions this week? ....

....

Other notes and observations about my training session or
my day ....

....

....

....

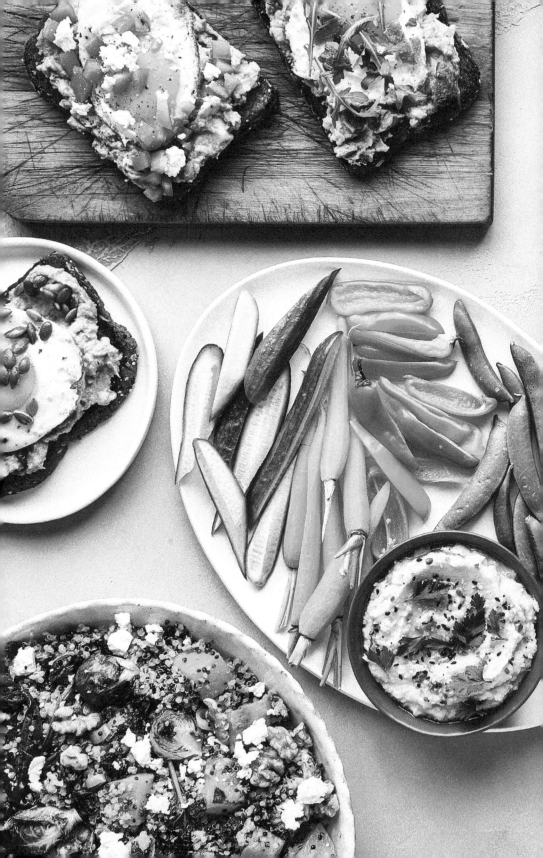

RECIPES

Since endurance is the product of total health and wellness, I want to help you get started with some easy recipes that incorporate the hero foods mentioned earlier in the book. If you can make mealtime easier, you'll have more success choosing foods that fuel your activities. With that in mind, I'm sharing recipes along with some tips for getting organized. These recipes are some of my family's favorites, and I hope you find they boost your health and overall performance.

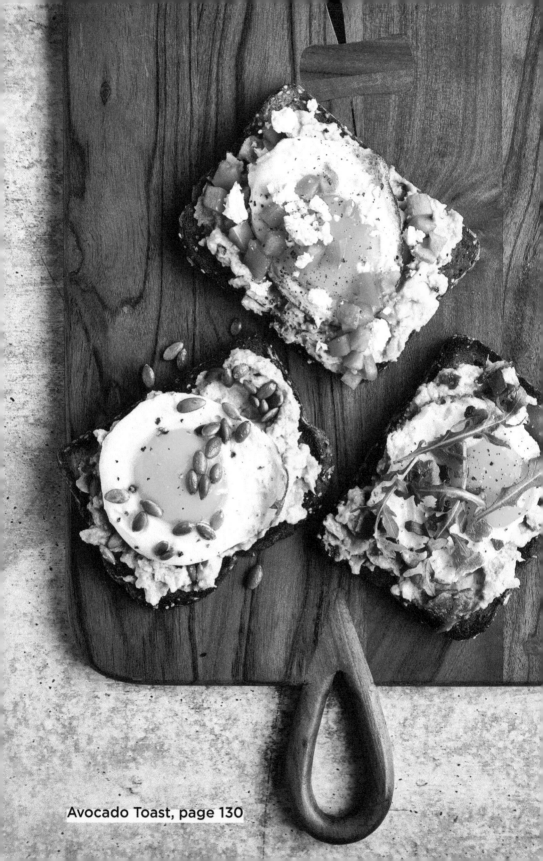

Avocado Toast, page 130

BREAKFAST

For breakfast, my focus is on make-ahead meals. Mornings can be hectic, but it's possible to start your day with a nutritious homemade meal.

Chia Pudding

SERVINGS 1 / PREP TIME 5 minutes / COOK TIME Refrigerate overnight

Chia pudding is the most fun to make in canning jars, but this is not a requirement. When I make this, I make enough for breakfast and snacks for the week.

INGREDIENTS

2 tablespoons chia seeds

½ banana, sliced, or ¼ cup sliced strawberries or blueberries

½ cup milk of your choice (almond milk, coconut milk, or banana milk)

INSTRUCTIONS

1. Combine the chia seeds, banana, and milk in a 1-pint canning jar. Stir gently.

2. Cover, and let sit in the refrigerator overnight.

TIP: To switch up the flavor, you can add in 1 tablespoon of peanut butter or a sprinkle of mini chocolate chips. My favorite variation is to swap the milk for Mooala Organic Chocolate Bananamilk.

Per Serving (using almond milk) Total Calories: 207; Total Fat: 10.4g; Sodium: 75.8mg; Total Carbohydrates: 27.5g; Fiber: 12g; Sugars: 10.7g; Protein: 7.1g

Overnight Oats

SERVINGS 1 / PREP TIME 5 minutes / COOK TIME Refrigerate overnight

This is another make-ahead canning-jar breakfast. Similar to chia pudding, these oats are refrigerated overnight, are served cold, and have a thick consistency. I prefer making my own oatmeal so I am in control of the amount and type of sugar I include, if any.

INGREDIENTS

½ cup rolled oats

½ cup milk, your choice

¼ cup sliced bananas, straw-berries, or blueberries

INSTRUCTIONS

1 Combine the oats, milk, and banana in a 1-pint canning jar. Stir gently.

2 Cover and let sit in the refrigerator overnight.

TIP: For a more traditional oatmeal, eliminate the fruit and add ¼ teaspoon of cinnamon and ½ teaspoon of vanilla extract.

ADDITIONAL OPTIONS: Using ½ cup of rolled oats and ½ cup of milk as the base, you can make other varieties.

CARROT CAKE: Add 1 teaspoon of shredded carrot, 1 tablespoon of raisins, 1 tablespoon of low-sugar vanilla yogurt, and 1 tablespoon of chopped almonds, pecans, or walnuts, in addition to the vanilla and cinnamon.

APPLE PIE: Add a quarter of an apple (chopped into small pieces), ¼ teaspoon of apple pie spice, and ½ teaspoon of vanilla extract.

Per Serving Total Calories: 214; Total Fat: 4.4g; Sodium: 75.5mg; Total Carbohydrates: 39.6g; Fiber: 5.5g; Sugars: 9.1g; Protein: 5.9g

Egg Cups

SERVINGS 12 / PREP TIME 15 minutes / COOK TIME 20 minutes

Egg cups are a portable, make-ahead favorite of mine for early mornings when I have family members running out of the house for school, work, and rehearsals. Pop these in the microwave for about 30 to 45 seconds, and you have a hot breakfast to go. Think of this as an omelet in muffin form. You can use any combination of fresh veggies, meats, and cheese.

INGREDIENTS

Nonstick cooking spray or 2 tablespoons olive oil

10 eggs

1 cup grated cheese

2 cups mixed sautéed vegetables such as onions, red peppers, spinach, or mushrooms

1 cup diced or shredded meat such as ham, chicken, or pork

Kosher salt

Freshly ground black pepper

INSTRUCTIONS

1 Preheat the oven to 350°F.

2 Spray a 12-cup muffin tin with cooking spray or wipe the bottom and sides with olive oil.

3 Crack the eggs into a bowl and mix until combined.

4 Spoon the cheese, vegetables, and meat into the muffin cups, filling no more than halfway up each cup.

5 Pour the egg mixture into each cup so each cup is three-fourths full.

6 Bake for 15 to 20 minutes, or until a toothpick inserted in the center comes out clean.

7 Refrigerate and use for quick meals and snacks throughout the week. Sprinkle with salt and pepper to taste before serving.

Per Serving (using sharp cheddar and diced chicken) Total Calories: 122; Total Fat: 7.9g; Sodium: 131.4mg; Total Carbohydrates: 1.3g; Fiber: 0.2g; Sugars: 0.5g; Protein: 10.9g

Pulled Pork Breakfast Tacos

SERVINGS 6 / PREP TIME 10 minutes / COOK TIME 10 to 15 minutes

This recipe takes a little prep, but it's super simple if you precook some shredded pork at the beginning of the week. For a make-ahead option, follow the recipe as directed. Then, wrap each breakfast taco in parchment paper and refrigerate them. You can heat individual tacos in the microwave for a quick breakfast option.

INGREDIENTS

6 eggs

1 cup cooked black beans

6 ounces pulled pork, previously prepared and seasoned with taco seasoning

Nonstick cooking spray

6 corn tortillas

½ cup salsa or diced tomatoes

1 avocado, sliced

1 cup shredded cheese (2 tablespoons per taco)

INSTRUCTIONS

1 Crack the eggs into a bowl and mix.

2 Cook the eggs in a nonstick pan over medium heat.

3 In separate pans, reheat the black beans and previously prepared pulled pork.

4 Lightly spray a pan with nonstick cooking spray and heat each tortilla.

5 Remove the tortillas from the pan, and add the cooked eggs, pork, black beans, salsa, avocado, and cheese to each taco before serving.

TIP: Prepare the pulled pork ahead of time in a slow cooker. Place a 3- to 5-pound pork shoulder in the slow cooker along with 1 cup of water and a packet of taco seasoning. Cook on low for 6 to 8 hours. Shred the meat with two forks.

Per Serving Total Calories: 372; Total Fat: 21.4g; Sodium: 389.3mg; Total Carbohydrates: 23.5g; Fiber: 5.7g; Sugars: 1.7g; Protein: 21.6g

Avocado Toast

SERVINGS 2 / PREP TIME 3 minutes / COOK TIME 5 minutes

My girls love avocado toast with a fried egg on top. You can use whole-grain bread, or if you prefer to go gluten-free, make your toast with Cauliflower Sandwich Thins from Outer Aisle.

INGREDIENTS

1 avocado

1 teaspoon kosher salt

1 teaspoon freshly ground black pepper

2 slices of bread, toasted

2 eggs, fried

Feta cheese, pepitas, diced tomatoes, bacon crumbles, arugula (all optional)

INSTRUCTIONS

1 Slice the avocado in half and remove the pit.

2 Scoop the avocado flesh into a bowl and mash it with a fork.

3 Sprinkle with kosher salt and freshly ground black pepper.

4 Spread the avocado onto the toast.

5 Place one fried egg on top of each toast.

OPTIONAL: If you want to get extra fancy, you can sprinkle feta cheese, pepitas, diced tomatoes, bacon crumbles, or arugula on top of the egg.

Per Serving Total Calories: 319; Total Fat: 19.6g; Sodium: 1351mg; Total Carbohydrates: 28.6g; Fiber: 10.1g; Sugars: 3.5g; Protein: 12.1g

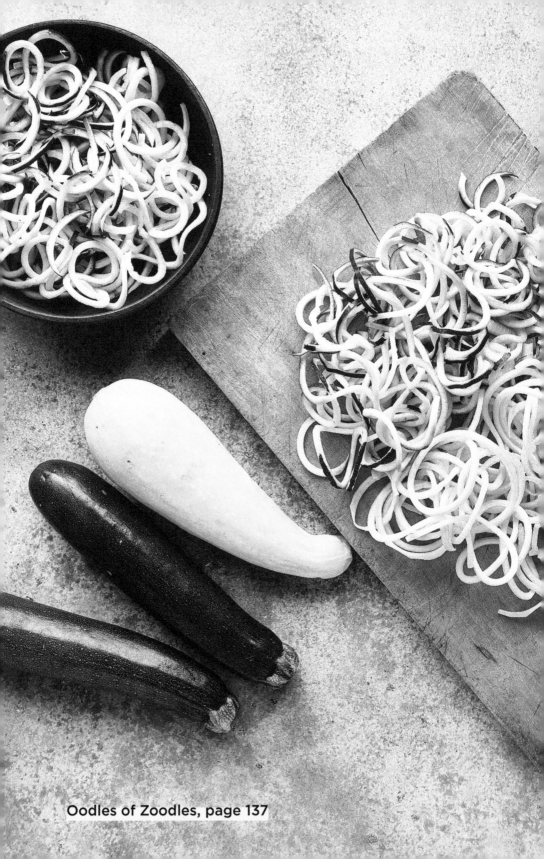

Oodles of Zoodles, page 137

LUNCH

Lunch calls for big-time meal prepping and planned leftovers. Rather than provide you with a bunch of recipes, I'm going to help you successfully plan and pack lunches that nourish. I have a collection of glass meal-prep containers with dividers and lids. (Google that exact phrase for dozens of options.) The containers make it easy to prep and store meals for the week.

Preparing your proteins in advance is the best tip I can give you. The first four recipes here are perfect to cook beforehand. You can do this over the weekend, or by cooking extra on nights you make time to prepare a full meal. I like to make shredded chicken, ground beef, hardboiled eggs, and quinoa to mix and match with lunches and dinners throughout the week.

Slow Cooker Shredded Chicken

SERVINGS 4 / PREP TIME 5 minutes / COOK TIME 6 to 8 hours

The slow cooker is my secret weapon for preparing nutritious meals when things get hectic around my house. Shredded chicken can add pizzazz to everything from salads to tacos, and cooking it ahead of time can mean the difference between another date with a takeout menu and a nutritious meal.

INGREDIENTS

4 chicken breasts

Kosher salt

Freshly ground black pepper

Garlic powder

Chicken broth

INSTRUCTIONS

1 Sprinkle the chicken breasts liberally with kosher salt, freshly ground black pepper, and garlic powder, and place them in the slow cooker with ½ inch of chicken broth filling the bottom of the cooker.

2 Cook on low for 6 to 8 hours. The chicken breasts should shred easily using two forks when done.

3 Separate the chicken into smaller portions, reserving some of the broth to keep it moist, and add seasonings to match your menu.

Per Serving Total Calories: 137; Total Fat: 3g; Sodium: 60.7mg; Total Carbohydrates: 0g; Fiber: 0g; Sugars: 0g; Protein: 25.7g

Perfect Hardboiled Eggs

SERVINGS 12 / PREP TIME 1 minute / COOK TIME 11 to 14 minutes

The perfect portable snack, and an easy protein to top off a salad or a piece of toast with, hardboiled eggs should be a staple. If you don't boil eggs often, it's easy to forget how long to cook them.

INGREDIENTS

12 eggs

INSTRUCTIONS

1 Place the eggs in the bottom of a pan in a single layer.

2 Add water to the pan, filling to 1 inch above the eggs.

3 Bring the water to a boil. Then take the pan off the heat and cover with a lid.

4 Set a timer for 11 to 14 minutes, cooking toward the top end of the range for firmer yolks.

5 When the timer goes off, place the pan under cold running water.

6 When the water in the pan is lukewarm, add ice cubes, and continue cooling the eggs for about 10 minutes. Refrigerate the eggs until you're ready to eat them.

Per Serving (per egg) Total Calories: 72; Total Fat: 4.8g; Sodium: 71mg; Total Carbohydrates: 0.4g; Fiber: 0g; Sugars: 0.2g; Protein: 6.3g

Spaghetti Squash Bowls

SERVINGS 2 to 4 / **PREP TIME** 2 minutes / **COOK TIME** 10 to 13 minutes

I love spaghetti squash all year round. When my family eats spaghetti, sloppy joes—anything with a sauce that is typically served on bread or noodles—I eat mine on top of spaghetti squash, zoodles, or rice noodles. Some people avoid spaghetti squash because they don't know how to cook it. I'm all for keeping things easy, so I cook mine in the microwave.

INGREDIENTS
1 spaghetti squash

INSTRUCTIONS

1 Wash the exterior of the spaghetti squash and use a knife to poke a few holes so the steam can escape.

2 Place the squash in the microwave for about 3 minutes, just long enough to soften the squash.

3 Cut the squash in half lengthwise, and use a spoon to scoop the seeds out.

4 Add ½ to 1 inch of water to a 9-by-13-inch glass baking dish, and place the squash in it face-down.

5 Cook in the microwave for 7 to 10 minutes (depending on the size of the squash and how your microwave cooks).

6 Use tongs to remove the squash from the baking dish. Using a fork, pull the strands from the shell toward the center of the squash. You will have strings of squash that look like spaghetti noodles.

7 Serve immediately, or store in a glass container in the refrigerator for up to 1 week.

TIP: If you're eating right away, there's no need to dirty any dishes. Just add your butter, seasonings, or sauces right to the squash "bowl" and enjoy!

Per Serving (per cup plain spaghetti squash) Total Calories: 42; Total Fat: 0.4g; Sodium: 27.9mg; Total Carbohydrates: 10g; Fiber: 2.2g; Sugars: 3.9g; Protein: 1g

Oodles of Zoodles

SERVINGS 1 to 2 per zucchini / PREP TIME 5 minutes / COOK TIME 10 minutes

Zoodles get their name because they are made from zucchini, but they can also be made from yellow squash. If you don't have a spiralizer, search for vegetable spiralizers online to see options. I'll admit I'm not always in the mood to make my own zoodles, so I buy premade zoodles in the prepared foods section at Whole Foods, on occasion.

INGREDIENTS

1 to 3 zucchini, depending on the number of people you are feeding

Butter

INSTRUCTIONS

1 Peel the zucchini, and use your vegetable spiralizer to create noodle-like strands.

2 In a large sauté pan or skillet, sauté the zoodles in a bit of organic butter until tender.

3 Eat immediately, or store in a container in the refrigerator and reheat later in the week.

Per Serving (per cup plain zucchini noodles) Total Calories: 20; Total Fat: 0.5g; Sodium: 10mg; Total Carbohydrates: 3.5g; Fiber: 1g; Sugars: 3g; Protein: 1.5g

Lunches to Prepare Now that You've Prepped

Once you have these recipes prepared, you can mix and match the food throughout the week as the base for the following creations.

Tacos and Taco Salad

When you prepare your meats for the week, add taco seasoning to at least half the mixture while it's still hot. When it's time to meal prep, portion one serving of meat into each glass meal-prep container you plan to use for Mexican-inspired meals. In the same container, add any other ingredients you plan to heat, such as black beans, rice, or quinoa. In a separate container, add lettuce, tomatoes, salsa, dressing, and any other cold items you like on your tacos or salads. When it's time to eat, microwave your container of items to be served hot and enjoy.

Spaghetti

Portion spaghetti squash, zoodles, or pasta noodles in your glass meal containers. On top of each pile of noodles, add a low-sugar marinara sauce and any of the meats you've prepared. Cover and store in the refrigerator until it's time to eat. Microwave prior to eating.

Salads

It's easy to consume a variety of fruits and vegetables when you think creatively about salads.

When jar salads were all the rage a few years ago, I found myself eating more salads because of the fun presentation, and incorporating more ingredients, helping me to eat the rainbow. Now I cut up fruits and veggies for the week and store them in a relish tray that has dividers and a lid. This becomes our at-home salad bar for the week, and I take it out each time salad will be served for a meal. If you don't want to chop veggies—or it's just you and you don't want a bunch of produce to go to waste—you can also purchase items like chopped cucumbers, shredded carrots, water chestnuts, artichoke hearts, and more from the salad bar at your grocery store.

If you plan to make a jar salad, the heaviest items, like meat or beans, go on the bottom, with lettuce going on the top. I prefer to keep the salad dressing separate, but you can also put it on the bottom of the jar.

Meat, Cheese, Egg, and Fruit Platter

It's so simple, it hardly seems like a meal. Sometimes, it's nice to pull out a container that takes you back to the day you enjoyed an antipasto platter in a cozy restaurant with a friend. Add a variety of cold meats, cheeses, fruits, olives, veggies with hummus, and hardboiled eggs. You can portion these in your meal-prep containers and pull them out for a quick lunch or snack.

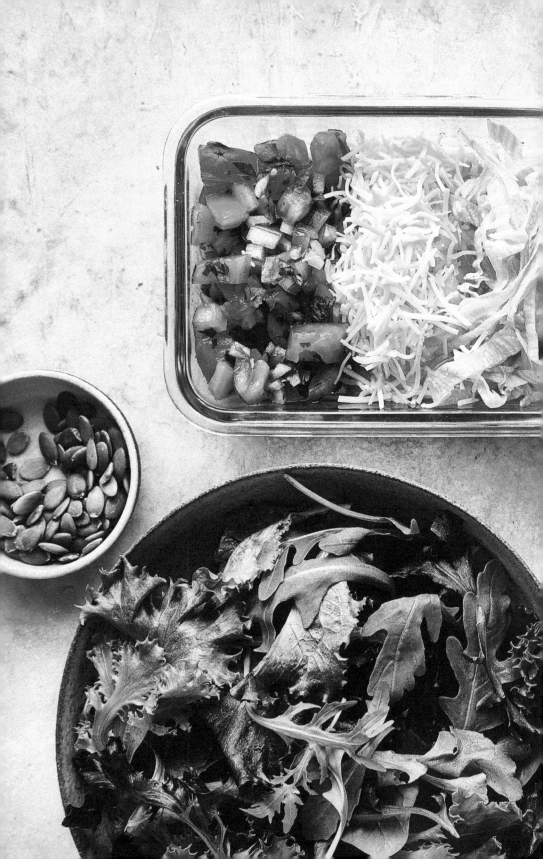

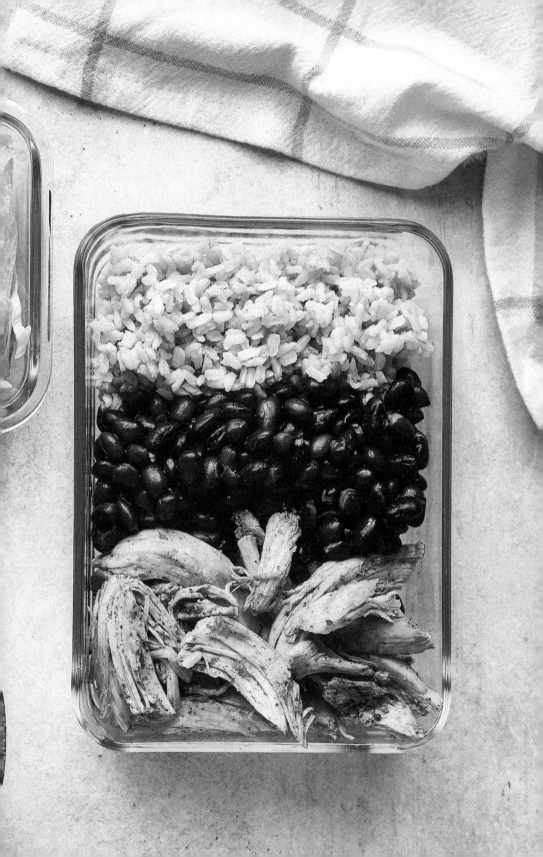

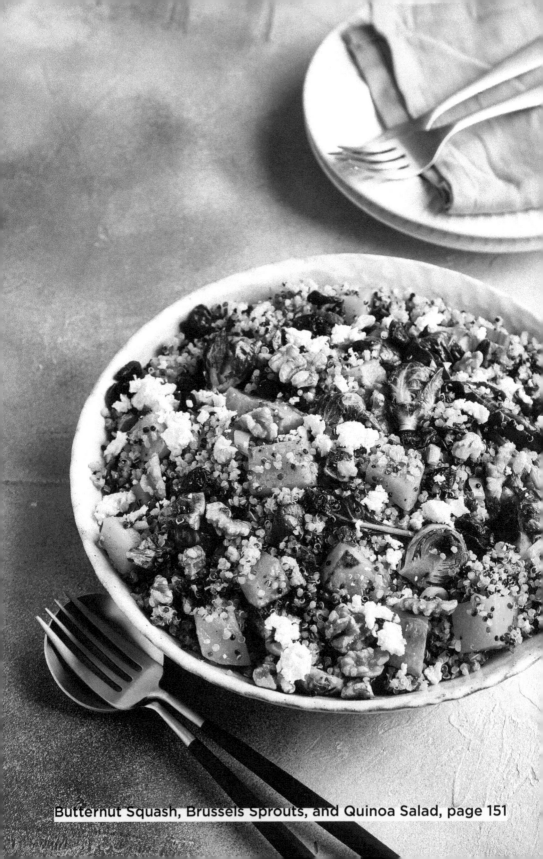

Butternut Squash, Brussels Sprouts, and Quinoa Salad, page 151

DINNER

The evening meal is usually when I take more time to cook. I often prepare food in the slow cooker while everyone is at work or school. Other nights, I have a hot meal ready for the first person to get home, and then I put the meal in the slow cooker on warm for other family members to eat as they come and go throughout the night. The following recipes include a combination of these methods. My goal is always to get my family to eat as many home-cooked meals as possible, which saves money and helps us consume fresh ingredients that are higher quality, with fewer preservatives and sugars than we'd typically get eating out.

Mexican Stuffed Peppers

SERVINGS 6 / PREP TIME 15 minutes / COOK TIME 40 minutes

This recipe brings back childhood memories of spending time in the kitchen with my mom. A comfort food, this meal comes together quickly if you've cooked any of the items earlier in the week.

INGREDIENTS

½ cup diced onions

½ pound ground turkey or beef, browned and seasoned with salt and freshly ground black pepper

4 cups cooked rice or quinoa, prepared according to package directions

1 (14-ounce) can diced, roasted tomatoes, drained

Taco seasoning packet

3 red, green, or yellow bell peppers, cut in half lengthwise with seeds and white parts removed

Shredded cheese, tomato salsa, and sour cream (all optional)

INSTRUCTIONS

1 Preheat the oven to 350°F.

2 In a sauté pan or skillet, sauté the onions.

3 Add the cooked meat, grains, roasted tomatoes, and taco seasoning. Stir to combine the ingredients until heated through.

4 Place the bell peppers open side up in a 9-by-13-inch baking dish with ½ inch of water in the bottom of the dish.

5 Fill the peppers with the skillet mixture.

6 Bake for 20 minutes.

OPTIONAL: Add shredded cheese the last 10 minutes and serve with tomato salsa and sour cream on top.

Per Serving (using 93% lean ground turkey) Total Calories: 255; Total Fat: 3.1g; Sodium: 660mg; Total Carbohydrates: 42.6g; Fiber: 3.3g; Sugars: 5.3g; Protein: 11.7g

Shredded Pork Taco Bowls

SERVINGS Makes 10 taco bowls / **PREP TIME** 10 minutes / **COOK TIME** 6 to 8 hours

It seems like we have a Mexican theme going on, but this one's another quick meal that I can count on my family to devour. As a bonus, the leftover meat tastes great on a salad, in an omelet, or in Egg Cups (page 128).

INGREDIENTS

3 to 5 pounds pork shoulder

1 packet taco seasoning

1 (15-ounce) can black beans, drained and rinsed

1 cup water, chicken broth, or vegetable broth

Mexican rice or quinoa, prepared according to package directions

TOPPINGS (OPTIONAL)

Tortilla chips

Shredded cheese

Tomato salsa

Sour cream

Shredded lettuce

INSTRUCTIONS

1 Place the pork shoulder in a slow cooker and pour the packet of taco seasoning on top.

2 Pour the beans on top of the pork.

3 Add the water or broth to the slow cooker.

4 Cover and cook on low for 6 to 8 hours.

5 Check to make sure the pork is 145°F before taking it out to shred. Using two forks, pull the forks away from each other.

6 Using a slotted spoon, scoop the beans out of the slow cooker, and add them to the shredded pork mixture.

7 Serve the pork mixture in bowls, adding the rice, cheese, salsa, and any additional toppings you like on tacos.

CONTINUED

TIP: I like to buy organic black beans in a can that is labeled BPA-free, and if I don't make my own seasoning, I use an organic seasoning packet. Prepare the rice or quinoa ahead of time to include in the taco bowls. We serve this with tortilla chips tucked along the edge of the bowl. For those sensitive to corn, a brand I love is Siete Grain-Free Tortilla Chips.

Per Serving Total Calories: 395; Total Fat: 27.5g; Sodium: 350.5mg; Total Carbohydrates: 8.8g; Fiber: 1.8g; Sugars: 1g; Protein: 25.2g

Individual Meat Loaves

SERVINGS 8 / PREP TIME 10 minutes / COOK TIME 20 minutes

I make these in an eight-cavity mini loaf pan because it's easy to serve and save in individual portions, plus tiny meat loaves cook faster and are just more fun.

INGREDIENTS

1 pound ground beef

1 cup brown rice bread crumbs, crushed crisp rice cereal, or bread crumb mixture

½ cup diced onion

½ cup diced red bell pepper

1 teaspoon garlic powder

½ teaspoon salt

½ teaspoon freshly ground black pepper

1 egg

Low-sugar barbecue sauce or ketchup

INSTRUCTIONS

1 Preheat the oven to 350°F.

2 Combine the beef, bread crumbs, onion, bell pepper, garlic powder, salt, black pepper, and egg in a large bowl and mix until incorporated.

3 Press the mixture into each loaf cavity, filling them three-quarters full.

4 Cook for about 20 minutes, or until the internal temperature is 145°F.

5 Before serving, top with a low-sugar barbecue sauce or ketchup.

Per Serving (using 90 percent lean ground beef) Total Calories: 167; Total Fat: 6.4g; Sodium: 424.9mg; Total Carbohydrates: 11.9g; Fiber: 0.9g; Sugars: 1.7g; Protein: 14.6g

Brussels Sprouts

SERVINGS 4 / PREP TIME 10 to 15 minutes / COOK TIME 20 minutes

We serve Brussels sprouts as a side dish at least once a week, and no one makes them as well as my daughter Katie, who created this recipe.

INGREDIENTS

12 ounces fresh Brussels sprouts

¼ cup white vinegar

2 tablespoons avocado oil or olive oil

2 teaspoons garlic powder, divided

½ teaspoon freshly ground black pepper, divided

½ teaspoon salt, divided

4 tablespoons butter

¼ teaspoon Italian seasoning

INSTRUCTIONS

1 Preheat the oven to 375°F.

2 Slice the hard end off of each sprout, slice in half lengthwise, and peel off any discolored leaves.

3 Place the sliced sprouts in a medium bowl, add the vinegar, and fill the bowl with water.

4 Let the sprouts soak for 2 to 5 minutes, then rinse them well. Pat them dry and place them in another medium bowl.

5 Add the oil to the bowl and mix, lightly coating each sprout.

6 Add 1 teaspoon of garlic powder, ¼ teaspoon of pepper, and ¼ teaspoon of salt, and stir.

7 Line a 10-by-15-inch baking sheet with parchment paper or aluminum foil and place the sprouts in a single layer.

8 Bake for 20 minutes. Keep an eye on the sprouts, because baking times will vary.

9 While the sprouts are cooking, in a medium bowl, combine the butter, Italian seasoning, and remaining 1 teaspoon of garlic powder, ¼ teaspoon of pepper, and ¼ teaspoon of salt, and beat with an electric mixer until the butter is a whipped consistency.

10 When the sprouts are done, spread the butter over them, and stir to coat.

Per Serving Total Calories: 209; Total Fat: 18.8g; Sodium: 394.2mg; Total Carbohydrates: 8.8g; Fiber: 3.4g; Sugars: 1.9g; Protein: 3.2g

Pizza Chicken

SERVINGS Makes 6 / **PREP TIME** 10 minutes / **COOK TIME** 15 to 20 minutes

This is my pizza of choice on a night when I'm not up for empty carbs. For an additional serving of veggies, include a salad.

INGREDIENTS

Nonstick cooking spray

3 chicken breasts

1 tablespoon avocado oil

1 (25-ounce) jar low-sugar marinara sauce

1 cup shredded provolone or mozzarella cheese

TOPPINGS (OPTIONAL)

Onions, diced

Peppers, diced

Olives, sliced

Pepperoni

Ham, diced

Any other toppings you would put on pizza

INSTRUCTIONS

1 Preheat the oven to 350°F.
2 Spray the bottom of a 9-by-13-inch glass baking dish with cooking spray.
3 Cut each chicken breast in half lengthwise.
4 In a large sauté pan or skillet, sauté the chicken in the oil until cooked through.
5 Place the chicken in the baking dish, and cover with marinara sauce. Add any toppings, and sprinkle cheese on top.
6 Bake for 5 to 7 minutes until the cheese is melted and the sauce is bubbly.

TIP: When you buy deli meats (such as pepperoni), look for meats that are free of nitrites, nitrates, and added sugars.

Per Serving Total Calories: 195; Total Fat: 9.5g; Sodium: 618.3mg; Total Carbohydrates: 9.2g; Fiber: 1.7g; Sugars: 5.8g; Protein: 17.8g

Butternut Squash, Brussels Sprouts, and Quinoa Salad

SERVINGS 6 / PREP TIME 30 minutes / COOK TIME 40 minutes

This colorful dish is great as a side or as a complete meal. I love the combination of colors, textures, and flavors. It reminds me of spending time in Savannah with my daughter Sarah—probably because I can't seem to get enough quinoa bowls when I visit her.

INGREDIENTS

1 medium butternut squash, peeled, seeded, and cubed

3 tablespoons avocado oil, divided

Kosher salt

Freshly ground black pepper

Garlic powder

2 cups baby spinach

1 cup uncooked quinoa

2 cups organic chicken broth or vegetable broth

1 clove garlic, diced

⅓ cup diced scallions

2 cups Brussels Sprouts (page 148)

½ cup dried, unsweetened cranberries

½ cup pumpkin seeds, sunflower seeds, or chopped walnuts

½ cup feta cheese

INSTRUCTIONS

1 Preheat the oven to 350°F.

2 Put the squash in a medium bowl and coat it with 2 tablespoons of oil.

3 Pour the squash onto a parchment- or foil-lined 10-by-15-inch baking sheet, sprinkle with salt, pepper, and garlic powder to taste, and cook for about 25 minutes, until a fork can easily penetrate the squash.

4 Take the squash out of the oven and allow to cool.

5 In a medium pot, combine the quinoa with the broth and bring to a boil.

6 Reduce the heat, cover, and cook on low for about 15 minutes, until the liquid is absorbed and the quinoa is tender.

CONTINUED

7   In a large sauté pan or skillet, sauté the garlic in the remaining 1 tablespoon of oil for about 1 minute, then add the scallions and spinach and cook until the spinach wilts.

8   In a large bowl, combine the squash, Brussels sprouts, quinoa, spinach mixture, cranberries, and pumpkin seeds.

9   Top each serving with feta cheese. Serve warm. Leftovers also taste amazing for breakfast with a fried egg on top.

Per Serving Total Calories: 339; Total Fat: 15g; Sodium: 480.2mg;

Total Carbohydrates: 42.8g; Fiber: 5.9g; Sugars: 11.4g; Protein: 9g

Baked Sweet Potato Slices

SERVINGS 4 to 6 / PREP TIME 10 to 15 minutes / COOK TIME 15 to 20 minutes

This is one of my favorite dishes on days when I'm hungry for fries but am listening to that voice that reminds me that my body doesn't need all the extra stuff that is in fast-food fries. My girls mastered this one early, and they each put their own spin on it.

INGREDIENTS

2 sweet potatoes, peeled and cut into ¼-inch slices

1 tablespoon avocado oil or olive oil

¼ teaspoon onion powder

¼ teaspoon garlic powder

¼ teaspoon salt

¼ teaspoon freshly ground black pepper

INSTRUCTIONS

1 Preheat the oven to 375°F.

2 Place the sweet potatoes in a medium bowl and lightly coat with the oil.

3 In a small bowl, combine the onion powder, garlic powder, salt, and pepper, and add the mixture to the bowl of potatoes. Stir to combine.

4 Place the potatoes on a parchment- or foil-lined 10-by-15-inch baking sheet in a single layer.

5 Bake for about 20 minutes. The cooking time will depend on the thickness of your slices, so check them often.

ADDITIONAL VARIATIONS: For a twist, add Parmesan cheese in the final 7 minutes of cooking, along with dried cranberries and precooked bacon crumbles. Another option is to prepare the sweet potatoes as described but cut them lengthwise to make thin slices. After you pull them out of the oven, top them with a fried egg and avocado slices, cream cheese and berries, peanut butter and banana, or your own combination of extras.

Per Serving Total Calories: 103; Total Fat: 3.7g; Sodium: 153.9mg; Total Carbohydrates: 16.2g; Fiber: 2g; Sugars: 2.7g; Protein: 1.2g

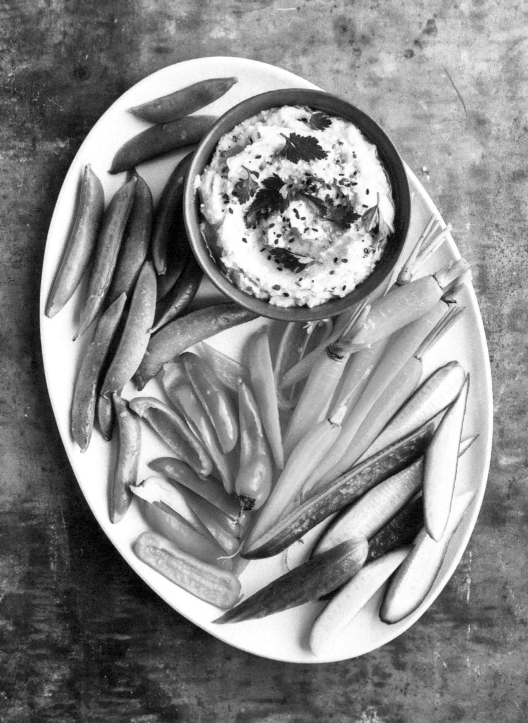

Everything Bagel Cauliflower Hummus, page 160

RESTORATIVE SNACKS

The recipes in this section can each work as a
nutritious snack or treat to share. Because
they are so flavorful, friends and family
members will gobble up these tasty treats.

Peanut Butter Energy Balls

SERVINGS 12 PREP TIME 5 minutes plus 40 minutes to chill

This recipe is an original from my friend Missy Malone, a runner I met in one of my Power of Run Facebook groups, who has become a great friend. Missy is a great cook, and she loves to run. She has the biggest heart and makes the most amazing personalized cards for every occasion.

INGREDIENTS

1 cup rolled oats

1 cup peanut butter

½ cup honey

1 cup shredded coconut

1 tablespoon chia seeds or flaxseed

1 teaspoon vanilla extract

1 tablespoon peanut butter protein powder

INSTRUCTIONS

1 In a large bowl, combine the oats, peanut butter, honey, coconut, chia seeds, vanilla, and protein powder.

2 Refrigerate until the mixture is firm, and then roll it into balls.

3 Store in a container in the refrigerator for up to a week.

Per Serving Total Calories: 249; Total Fat: 15.1g; Sodium: 122.3mg; Total Carbohydrates: 25.7g; Fiber: 3.1g; Sugars: 14.1g; Protein: 7.4g

Trail Mix

Everybody loves a good trail mix. It's an easy snack for days when you're on the go. While nuts are highly nutritious, they are also high in calories, so watch your portion sizes.

INGREDIENTS

1 cup cashews

1 cup almonds

1 cup macadamia nuts

¼ cup shredded coconut

¼ cup dried cranberries or raisins

INSTRUCTIONS

In a large bowl, mix together the cashews, almonds, macadamia nuts, coconut, and cranberries. Store in an airtight container.

> TIP: When buying dried fruits, look for an option without sugar or sweetener added. If you're in the mood for something a little sweeter, add a few white chocolate chips—they taste great with cranberries!

Per Serving Total Calories: 350; Total Fat: 30.6g; Sodium: 11.1mg; Total Carbohydrates: 16.5g; Fiber: 4.5g; Sugars: 4.8g; Protein: 8g

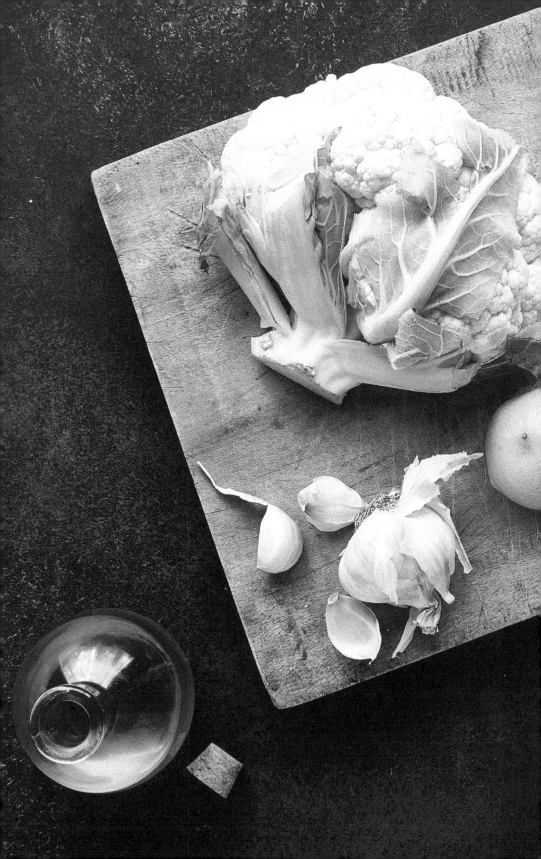

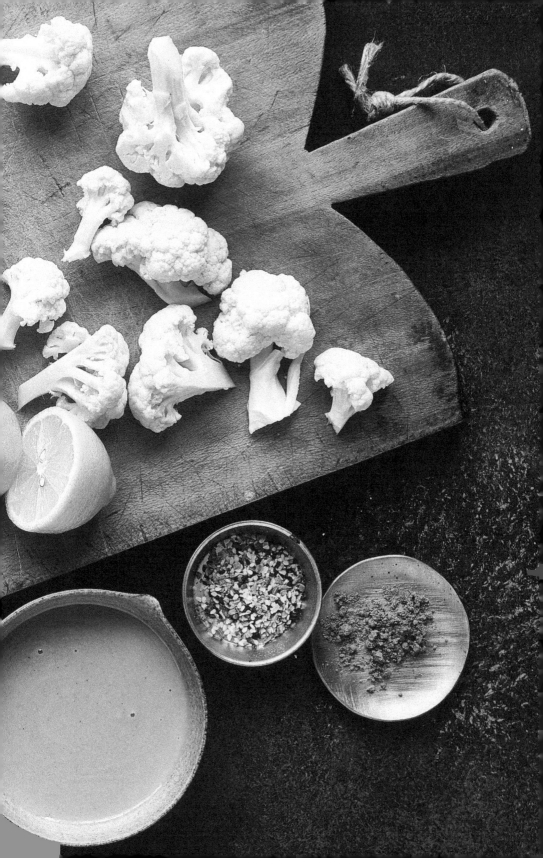

Everything Bagel Cauliflower Hummus

I can't be the only one who could eat hummus by the spoonful. I created this hummus so I could consume generous portions of it with my veggies. This recipe uses steamed cauliflower instead of the traditional garbanzo beans. Use this as a dip for snap peas, cucumbers, carrots, peppers, or celery.

INGREDIENTS

1 medium head cauliflower

3 tablespoons olive oil or avocado oil

2 tablespoons tahini (a paste made of ground sesame seeds, usually found next to the nut butters or in the ethnic foods aisle)

2 tablespoons freshly squeezed lemon juice

1 garlic clove

1 tablespoon Everything Bagel Seasoning (widely available at grocery stores or online)

¼ teaspoon salt

½ teaspoon ground cumin

Olive oil, sunflower seeds, sliced olives, and fresh parsley leaves (optional, all for garnish)

INSTRUCTIONS

1 Cut the florets from the head of the cauliflower. In a large pot with the cover on over medium heat, steam the cauliflower in 1 cup of water until it is tender.

2 Strain the cauliflower in a colander and use paper towels to press out any extra liquid.

3 In a food processor, combine the cauliflower, oil, tahini, lemon juice, garlic, Everything Bagel Seasoning, salt, and cumin. Blend until all the ingredients are combined and the mixture is a smooth texture.

4 Place in a glass container with a lid and store in the refrigerator for up to 1 week.

5 Add garnishes before serving.

Per Batch Total Calories: 757; Total Fat: 62.7g; Sodium: 1,757mg;

Total Carbohydrates: 39.7g; Fiber: 17.5g; Sugars: 11.6g; Protein: 17g

Avocado Chicken Salad Bites

SERVINGS 6 / PREP TIME 10 minutes

Is there anything better than avocado, chicken, and hardboiled eggs? I love this recipe because it's so versatile: It can be a meal, a snack, or even an appetizer. And, the salad does not need to be confined to a tortilla.

INGREDIENTS

2 cups chicken, cooked and shredded

1 avocado, mashed

2 tablespoons mayonnaise (use real mayo)

1½ tablespoons freshly squeezed lime juice

2 tablespoons diced scallions

2 hardboiled eggs, mashed

¼ teaspoon salt

½ teaspoon garlic powder

6 large flour tortillas

INSTRUCTIONS

1 In a large bowl, combine the chicken, avocado, mayonnaise, lime juice, scallions, eggs, salt, and garlic powder, and mix together.

2 Spread the mixture onto the tortillas.

3 Roll the tortillas, and slice them into 1-inch bites.

TIP: For an extra serving of veggies, you can opt to serve the mixture stuffed in halved baby bell peppers. Cut the baby peppers in half lengthwise and scoop out the seeds and pulp. Add heaping portions of the salad to the pepper halves.

Per Serving (using 10-inch tortillas) Total Calories: 427; Total Fat: 18.2g; Sodium: 516.9mg; Total Carbohydrates: 43.1g; Fiber: 4.5g; Sugars: 0.9g; Protein: 21.8g

Parmesan Zucchini Fries

SERVINGS 3 / PREP TIME 20 minutes / COOK TIME 25 minutes

The pork rinds add a surprising amount of protein to this dish. With a little shredded chicken on top, you'll forget you're eating zucchini fries instead of French fries.

INGREDIENTS

2½ ounces all-natural pork rinds, crushed into crumbs (or 2 cups bread crumbs)

¾ cup Parmesan cheese, grated, divided

2 eggs

2 small zucchini, cut into strips

INSTRUCTIONS

1 Preheat the oven to 350°F.

2 Pour the pork rind crumbs into a medium bowl and add ½ cup of Parmesan cheese.

3 In a separate medium bowl, crack and mix the eggs.

4 Pour a small amount of the crumb mixture onto a plate.

5 Dip the zucchini strips in the egg mixture, then roll them in the crumb mixture, pressing the crumbs and cheese into the zucchini.

6 Place each slice on a 10-by-15-inch baking sheet lined with parchment paper or aluminum foil.

7 Continue working in small batches, adding more crumbs as needed. Avoid dumping the entire bag of crumbs onto the plate; you will wind up with a pile of wet crumbs, which won't stick well to the zucchini.

8 Bake for 25 minutes, using tongs to gently flip the fries half-way through. Sprinkle them with the remaining ¼ cup of Parmesan cheese during the last 5 minutes of baking.

Per Serving Total Calories: 304; Total Fat: 19.7g; Sodium: 455.3mg; Total Carbohydrates: 3.9g; Fiber: 0.9g; Sugars: 1.5g; Protein: 29.1g

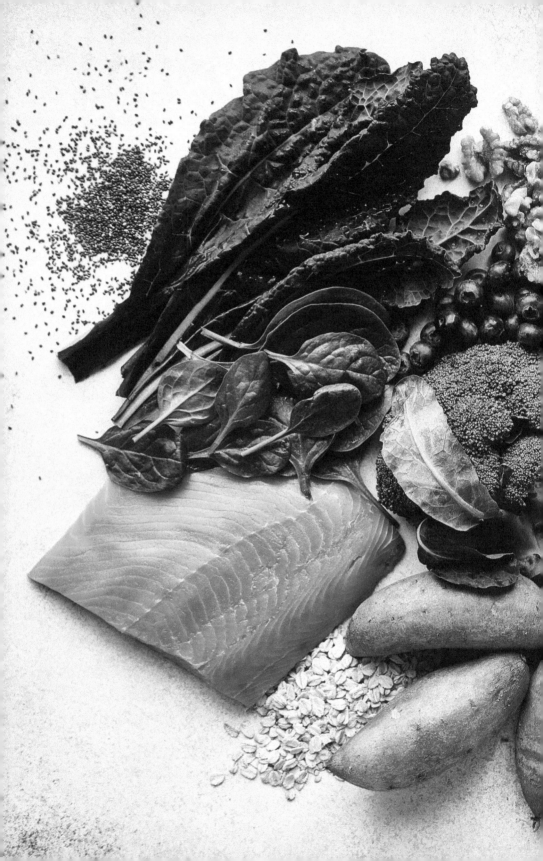

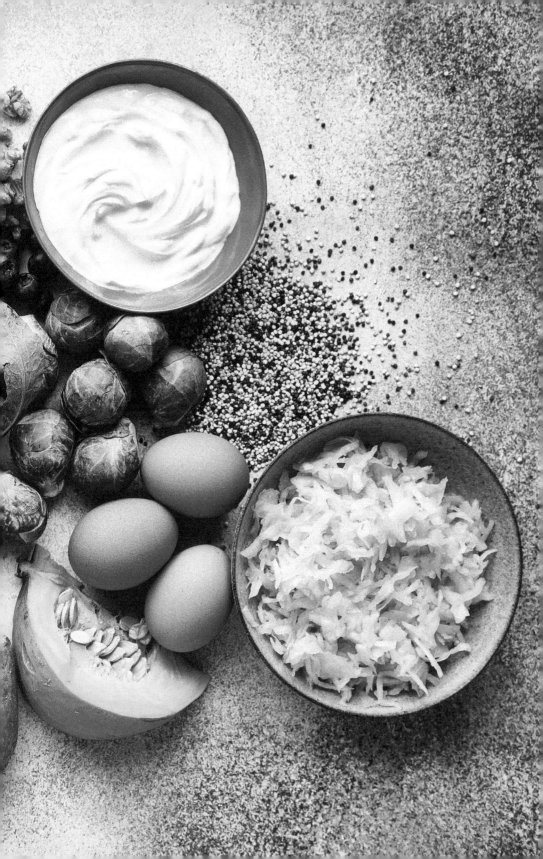

RESOURCES

Books

Anatomy for Runners: Unlocking Your Athletic Potential for Health, Speed, and Injury Prevention by Jay Dicharry, MPT, SCS—This book should be every athlete's guide to running injury-free. Another one of Jay's books, *Running Rewired: Reinvent Your Run for Stability, Strength, and Speed*, should also be at the top of every runner's list.

Atomic Habits: An Easy & Proven Way to Build Good Habits & Break Bad Ones by James Clear—With tips and techniques for creating positive habits and eliminating habits that don't serve you, this book is a must-read for any athlete who struggles to create behavior change that sticks.

Finding Your Sweet Spot: How to Avoid RED-S (Relative Energy Deficit in Sport) by Optimizing Your Energy Balance by Rebecca McConville, MS, RD, CSSD, CEDRD—This book explains RED-S in detail and helps athletes understand the warning signs and causes, how to find balance, and how to prevent or recover from RED-S.

Let Your Mind Run: A Memoir of Thinking My Way to Victory by Deena Kastor—If you want to learn to harness the power of your mind while also reading the story about how Deena Kastor used optimism to become one of the greatest elite athletes of our time, you need this book.

ROAR: How to Match Your Food and Fitness to Your Female Physiology for Optimum Performance, Great Health, and a Strong, Lean Body for Life by Stacy T. Sims, PhD—This book is an eye-opening look at the ways women should train and nourish their bodies differently than men.

Run for Your Life: How to Run, Walk, and Move Without Pain or Injury and Achieve a Sense of Well-Being and Joy by Mark Cucuzzella, MD—Dr. Cucuzzella is a leading expert in all things healthy running, and in this book, he explains everything a runner would want to know about biomechanics, nutrition, and running injury-free.

Podcasts

Search your favorite podcast app for each of these podcasts:

Couch to Active—Lyn Lindbergh, author of the award-winning book *Couch to Active: The Missing Link that Takes You from Sedentary to Active*, helps listeners get off the couch and exercise in a way that helps them smile.

Phit for a Queen—Created by Rebecca McConville, MS, RD, CSSD, CEDRD, and Kara Shelman, LCSW, MPH, this podcast is devoted to female athletes wanting to have it all: performance health, intellect, and time for self.

Power Up Your Performance—This one is my own podcast. With a focus on helping people learn to think, feel, perform, and live like champions, I cover mind-set, wellness, and endurance topics each week.

Online

Clean Sport Collective—This is a community of powerful voices including athletes, brands, events, clubs, fans, and the public to support the pursuit of clean sports and athletics through the absence of performance-enhancing drugs. *https://cleansport.org/*

Heather Denniston, DC, CCWP—*The Junk You Should Know Show*—Dr. Denniston is a seasoned chiropractor, speaker, athlete, health enthusiast, and writer who has a passion for inspiring people of all ages to take the first steps toward realizing their greatness. She offers a weekly show each Friday, available from her Facebook page or website, that covers wellness topics in 30 minutes. *https://www.wellfitandfed.com/the-official-junk-you-should-know-show*

Dina Griffin, MS, RDN, CSSD, CISSN, METS II—The Nutrition Mechanic—Dina offers an online endurance nutrition primer for athletes of all abilities. Her program is an excellent source for athletes who would like help with daily nutrition and race-day fueling. *https://nutritionmechanic.com/*

James O'Keefe, MD—"Run for Your Life!" (TEDx Talk)—Dr. O'Keefe is a cardiologist and "medical director of the Saint Luke's Charles & Barbara Duboc Cardio Health & Wellness Center at the Mid America Heart Institute in Kansas City, Missouri. He is actively involved in research and presented this TEDx Talk about the possible dangers of excessive exercise. You can view this talk at *https://youtu.be/Y6U728AZnV0*. I include his other talks in a playlist available on my website.

Dr. Emily Splichal, DPM—Dr. Splichal is a human movement specialist and a global leader in barefoot science and foot rehabilitation. She has a wealth of resources that you can access via her website. Be sure to click through to her YouTube playlist, which contains educational videos for running injury-free. *https://www.dremilysplichal.com/*

Governing Body Websites

National Collegiate Athletic Association (NCAA)—Doping and Substance Abuse homepage. *http://www.ncaa.org/sport -science-institute/alcohol-and-other-recreational-drug-prevention*

USA Cycling—The national governing body for cycling in the United States. Get news, updates of rules, and athlete resources. *https://www.usacycling.org/*

USA Swimming—The national governing body for the sport of swimming in the United States. Get news, updates of rules, and athlete resources. *https://www.usaswimming.org/*

USA Track and Field—The national governing body for track and field. Get news, updates of rules, and athlete resources. *http:// www.usatf.org/*

USA Triathlon—The national governing body for triathlon in the United States. Get news, updates of rules, and athlete resources. *https://www.teamusa.org/usa-triathlon*

US Olympic Committee—Team USA Athlete Services Nutrition Page. On this site, you can access the Athlete's Plates and all the USOC nutrition resources referred to in this book. *https://www .teamusa.org/nutrition*

US Rowing—The national governing body for the sport of rowing in the United States. Get news, updates of rules, and athlete resources. *https://usrowing.org/*

Visit my website, *https://www.crushingmygoals.com*, for links to all these resources.

REFERENCES

Chapter One

"Is Endurance Training Bad for You? Sports Medicine Physicians Find No Evidence of Heart Damage from Long-Term Endurance Training by Elite Master Athletes." *ScienceDaily*, May 31, 2016. https://www.sciencedaily.com/releases/2016/05/160531104518.htm.

Centers for Disease Control and Prevention. "Lack of Physical Activity." September 25, 2019. https://www.cdc.gov/chronicdisease/resources/publications/factsheets/physical-activity.htm.

O'Keefe, James H. "Run for Your Life! At a Comfortable Pace, and Not Too Far." *TEDxUMKC*. Uploaded November 27, 2012. https://youtu.be/Y6U728AZnV0.

O'Keefe, James H., Evan L. O'Keefe, and Carl J. Lavie. "The Goldilocks Zone for Exercise: Not Too Little, Not Too Much." *Missouri Medicine* 115, no. 2 (March/April 2018): 98–104. https://www.ncbi.nlm.nih.gov/pmc/articles/PMC6139866/pdf/ms115_p0098.pdf.

O'Keefe, James H., Harshal R. Patil, Carl J. Lavie, Anthony Magalski, Robert A. Vogel, and Peter A. McCullough. "Potential Adverse Cardiovascular Effects from Excessive Endurance Exercise." *Mayo Clinic Proceedings* 87, no. 6 (June 2012): 587–95. https://www.ncbi.nlm.nih.gov/pmc/articles/PMC3538475/.

Turnwald, Bradley P., J. Parker Goyer, Danielle Z. Boles, Amy Silder, Scott L. Delp, and Alia J. Crum. "Learning One's Genetic Risk Changes Physiology Independent of Actual Genetic Risk." *Nature Human Behaviour* 3 (2019): 48–56. https://www.nature.com/articles/s41562-018-0483-4.

Wilcock, Bob. "The 1908 Olympic Marathon." *Journal of Olympic History* 16, no. 1 (March 2008): 31–47. http://isoh.org/wp-content/uploads/2015/03/177.pdf.

Chapter Two

Byrd, Bryant R., Jamie Keith, Shawn M. Keeling, Ryan M. Weatherwax, Paul B. Nolan, Joyce S. Ramos, and Lance C. Dalleck. "Personalized Moderate-Intensity Exercise Training Combined with High-Intensity Interval Training Enhances Training Responsiveness." *International Journal of Environmental Research and Public Health* 16, no. 12 (June 2019): 2088. https://doi.org/10.3390/ijerph16122088.

Cain, Mary. "I Was the Fastest Girl in America, Until I Joined Nike." *New York Times*, November 7, 2019. https://www.nytimes.com/2019/11/07/opinion/nike-running-mary-cain.html.

Emmons, Robert. "Why Gratitude Is Good." *Greater Good Magazine*, November 16, 2010. https://greatergood.berkeley.edu/article/item/why_gratitude_is_good/.

Stöggl, Thomas, and Billy Sperlich. "Polarized Training Has Greater Impact on Key Endurance Variables Than Threshold, High Intensity, or High Volume Training." *Frontiers in Physiology* 5, no. 33 (February 2014). https://doi.org/10.3389/fphys.2014.00033.

US Anti-Doping Agency. "AAA Panel Imposes 4-Year Sanctions on Alberto Salazar and Dr. Jeffrey Brown for Multiple Anti-Doping Rule Violations." September 30, 2019. https://www.usada.org/sanction/aaa-panel-4-year-sanctions-alberto-salazar-jeffrey-brown/.

Chapter Three

Ballantyne, Sarah. "5 Nutrients You're Deficient In . . . If You Eat Too Much Sugar." The Paleo Mom website. December 5, 2015. https://www.thepaleomom.com/5-nutrients-youre-deficient-in-if-you-eat-too-much-sugar/.

Black, David S., and George M. Slavich. "Mindfulness Meditation and the Immune System: A Systematic Review of Randomized Controlled Trials." *Annals of the New York Academy of Sciences* 1373, no. 1 (June 2016): 13–24. https://doi.org/10.1111/nyas.12998.

Bradley University. "Eating Disorders: Orthorexia." https://www.bradley.edu/sites/bodyproject/disorders/orthorexia/.

DiNicolantonio, James J., and Amy Berger. "Added Sugars Drive Nutrient and Energy Deficit in Obesity: A New Paradigm." *Open Heart* 3, no. 2 (August 2016). http://dx.doi.org/10.1136/openhrt-2016-000469.

Guest, Nanci S., Justine Horne, Shelley M. Vanderhout, and Ahmed El-Sohemy. "Sport Nutrigenomics: Personalized Nutrition for Athletic Performance." *Frontiers in Nutrition* 6, no. 8 (February 2019). https://doi.org/10.3389/fnut.2019.00008.

Harvard T. H. Chan School of Public Health. "Doctors Need More Nutrition Education." 2017. https://www.hsph.harvard.edu/news/hsph-in-the-news/doctors-nutrition-education/.

Harvard T. H. Chan School of Public Health. "Healthy Eating Plate." https://www.hsph.harvard.edu/nutritionsource/healthy-eating-plate/.

Lenoir, Magalie, Fuschia Serre, Lauriane Cantin, and Serge H. Ahmed. "Intense Sweetness Surpasses Cocaine Reward." *PLOS ONE*. August 1, 2007. https://doi.org/10.1371/journal.pone.0000698.

Martínez Steele, Eurídice, Larissa Galastri Baraldi, Maria Laura da Costa Louzada, Jean-Claude Moubarac, Dariush Mozaffarian, and Carlos Augusto Monteiro. "Ultra-Processed Foods and Added Sugars in the US Diet: Evidence from a Nationally Representative Cross-Sectional Study." *BMJ Open* 6, no. 3 (March 2016). http://dx.doi.org/10.1136/bmjopen-2015-009892.

McConville, Rebecca. *Finding Your Sweet Spot: How to Avoid RED-S (Relative Energy Deficit in Sport) by Optimizing Your Energy Balance.* Published independently, 2019.

Moore, Evan. "CoachCast: Optimizing Physiology with Stacy Sims." *TrainingPeaks Coach Blog.* Episode 22, June 5, 2019. https://www.trainingpeaks.com/coach-blog/coachcast-optimizing-physiology-with-stacy-sims/.

Nettleton, Jennifer A., Pamela L. Lutsey, Youfa Wang, João A. Lima, Erin D. Michos, and David R. Jacobs, Jr. "Diet Soda Intake and Risk of Incident Metabolic Syndrome and Type 2 Diabetes in the Multi-Ethnic Study of Atherosclerosis (MESA)." *Diabetes Care* 32, no. 4 (April 2009): 688–94. https://doi.org/10.2337/dc08-1799.

Ng, Shu Wen, Meghan M. Slining, and Barry M. Popkin. "Use of Caloric and Noncaloric Sweeteners in US Consumer Packaged Foods, 2005-2009." *Journal of the Academy of Nutrition and Dietetics* 112, no. 11 (November 2012): 1828–34. https://doi.org/10.1016/j.jand.2012.07.009.

Parr, Evelyn B., Donny M. Camera, José L. Areta, Louise M. Burke, Stuart M. Phillips, John A. Hawley, and Vernon G. Coffey. "Alcohol Ingestion Impairs Maximal Post-Exercise Rates of Myofibrillar Protein Synthesis Following a Single Bout of Concurrent Training." *PLOS ONE*, February 12, 2014. https://doi.org/10.1371/journal.pone.0088384.

Peek, Kim. "Mark Cucuzzella: On Nutrition, Running, and Fast Shoes." *Power Up Your Performance.* Podcast, episode 80, November 12, 2019. https://powerup.libsyn.com/mark-cucuzzella-on-nutrition-running-and-fast-shoes.

Sandoiu, Ana. "Just 20 Minutes of Exercise Enough to Reduce Inflammation, Study Finds." *Medical News Today*, January 16, 2017. https://www.medicalnewstoday.com/articles/315255.php.

Sims, Stacy. "Women Are Not Small Men: A Paradigm Shift in the Science of Nutrition." *TEDxTauranga.* Uploaded September 23, 2019. https://youtu.be/e5LYGzKUPlE.

Strawbridge, Holly. "Artificial Sweeteners: Sugar-Free, but at What Cost?" *Harvard Health* (blog). January 8, 2018. https://www.health .harvard.edu/blog/artificial-sweeteners-sugar-free-but-at-what -cost-201207165030.

Team USA. "Nutrition." https://www.teamusa.org/nutrition.

Thebe, Amanda. "Dr Stacy Sims Talks Menopause." *Fit & Chips Chats with Amanda Thebe*. Podcast, episode 50. https://www.fitnchips.com/ 2019/04/dr-stacy-sims-talks-menopause/.

University of California San Francisco. "Hidden in Plain Sight: Added Sugar Is Hiding in 74% of Packaged Foods." SugarScience website. http://sugarscience.ucsf.edu/hidden-in-plain-sight/#.XZ3-xEZKjLY.

University of California San Francisco. "How Much Is Too Much? The Growing Concern over Too Much Added Sugar in Our Diets." Sugar-Science website. https://sugarscience.ucsf.edu/the-growing-concern -of-overconsumption.html#.Xb4hbppKjLZ.

United States Olympic Committee. "USOC Sports Nutrition Alcohol Factsheet." https://www.teamusa.org/nutrition.

University of East Anglia. "Eating Blueberries Every Day Improves Heart Health." *ScienceDaily*. May 30, 2019. https://www.sciencedaily .com/releases/2019/05/190530101221.htm.

US Food & Drug Administration. "Spilling the Beans: How Much Caffeine Is Too Much?" December 12, 2018. https://www.fda.gov/ consumers/consumer-updates/spilling-beans-how-much-caffeine -too-much/.

Chapter Four

Bachus, Tiffani, and Erin Macdonald. "How to Eat and Train for a Mesomorph Body Type." American Council on Exercise website. September 18, 2014. https://www.acefitness.org/education-and -resources/lifestyle/blog/5039/how-to-eat-and-train-for-a -mesomorph-body-type.

Bachus, Tiffani, and Erin Macdonald. "How to Eat and Train for an Ectomorph Body Type." American Council on Exercise website. October 3, 2014. https://www.acefitness.org/education-and-resources/lifestyle/blog/5102/how-to-eat-and-train-for-an-ectomorph-body-type.

Bachus, Tiffani, and Erin Macdonald. "How to Eat and Train for an Endomorph Body Type." American Council on Exercise website. September 26, 2014. https://www.acefitness.org/education-and-resources/lifestyle/blog/5078/how-to-eat-and-train-for-an-endomorph-body-type.

Gowery, Dawn. "Oxytocin: The Hormone of Love and Trust." *Healthy Beginnings Lifestyle Magazine*. May 1, 2015. https://hbmag.com/20637-2/.

Keay, Nicky. "2018 UPDATE: Relative Energy Deficiency in Sport (RED-S)." *British Journal of Sports Medicine* (blog). May 30, 2018. https://blogs.bmj.com/bjsm/2018/05/30/2018-update-relative-energy-deficiency-in-sport-red-s/.

McConville, Rebecca. *Finding Your Sweet Spot: How to Avoid RED-S (Relative Energy Deficit in Sport) by Optimizing Your Energy Balance*. Published independently, 2019.

Payne, Andrew. "Body Types: How to Train and Diet for Your Body Type." NASM website. May 28, 2019. https://blog.nasm.org/fitness/body-types-how-to-train-diet-for-your-body-type/.

Chapter Five

Angus, Simon D. "A Statistical Timetable for the Sub–2-Hour Marathon." *Medicine & Science in Sports & Exercise* 51, no. 7 (July 2019): 1460–6. doi:10.1249/MSS.0000000000001928.

Beresini, Erin. "How Long Should I Hold a Stretch?" Outside Online. https://www.outsideonline.com/1783541/how-long-should-i-hold-stretch.

Moller, Lorraine. "Hill Training—The Lydiard Way." Lydiard Foundation. https://lydiardfoundation.org/hill-training-the-lydiard-way/.

National Sleep Foundation. "How Sleep Affects Athletes' Performance: Find Out Why Snoozing More Will Keep You on Top of Your Game." Sleep.org. https://www.sleep.org/articles/how-sleep-affects-athletes/.

Peek, Kim. "Mark Cucuzzella: On Nutrition, Running, and Fast Shoes." *Power Up Your Performance.* Podcast, episode 80, November 12, 2019. https://powerup.libsyn.com/mark-cucuzzella-on-nutrition-running-and-fast-shoes.

Quealy, Kevin, and Josh Katz. "Nike Says Its $250 Running Shoes Will Make You Run Much Faster. What If That's Actually True?" *New York Times.* July 18, 2019. https://www.nytimes.com/interactive/2018/07/18/upshot/nike-vaporfly-shoe-strava.html?module=inline.

Robinson, Justin. "Overtraining: 9 Signs of Overtraining to Look Out For." American Council on Exercise website. June 21, 2017. https://www.acefitness.org/education-and-resources/lifestyle/blog/6466/overtraining-9-signs-of-overtraining-to-look-out-for.

Chapter Six

Blanchfield, A. W., J. Hardy, H. M. De Morree, W. Staiano, and S. M. Marcora. "Talking Yourself Out of Exhaustion: The Effects of Self-Talk on Endurance Performance." *Medicine & Science in Sports & Exercise* 46, no. 5 (May 2014): 998–1007. doi:10.1249/MSS.0000000000000184.

Di Rienzo, Franck, Ursula Debarnot, Sébastien Daligault, Elodie Saruco, Claude Delpuech, Julien Doyon, Christian Collet, and Aymeric Guillot. "Online and Offline Performance Gains Following Motor Imagery Practice: A Comprehensive Review of Behavioral and Neuroimaging Studies." *Frontiers in Human Neuroscience.* June 28, 2016. https://doi.org/10.3389/fnhum.2016.00315.

Jahnke, Roger, Linda Larkey, Carol Rogers, Jennifer Etnier, and Fang Lin. "A Comprehensive Review of Health Benefits of Qigong and Tai Chi." *American Journal of Health Promotion* 24, no. 6 (July–August 2010): e1–e25. doi:10.4278/ajhp.081013-LIT-248.

Korb, Alex. "The Grateful Brain: The Neuroscience of Giving Thanks." *Psychology Today.* November 20, 2012. https://www.psychologytoday .com/us/blog/prefrontal-nudity/201211/the-grateful-brain.

National Athletic Trainers' Association. "National Athletic Trainers' Association Releases Official Statement of Recommendations to Reduce the Risk of Injury Related to Sport Specialization for Adolescent and Young Athletes." October 16, 2019. https://www.newswise .com/articles/national-athletic-trainers-association-releases-official -statement-of-recommendations-to-reduce-the-risk-of-injury -related-to-sport-specialization-for-adolescent-and-young-athletes.

National Qigong Association. http://www.nqa.org/.

Peek, Kim. "BONUS: Boston Marathon Celebration of Champions." *Power Up Your Performance.* Podcast, April 14, 2019. http://powerup .libsyn.com/bonus-boston-marathon-celebration-of-champions.

Peek, Kim. "Thinking Her Way to Victory with Deena Kastor." *Power Up Your Performance.* Podcast, episode 53, May 21, 2019. https://powerup .libsyn.com/53-thinking-her-way-to-victory-with-deena-kastor.

Peek, Kim. "What It Takes to Crush Your Goals." *Power Up Your Performance.* Podcast, episode 50, April 30, 2019. https://powerup.libsyn .com/nick-symmonds-talks-running-training-goals-and-pursuing -your-dreams.

Ranganathan, Vinoth K., Vlodek Siemionow, Jing Z. Liu, Vinod Sahgal, and Guang H. Yue. "From Mental Power to Muscle Power—Gaining Strength by Using the Mind." *Neuropsychologia* 42, no. 7 (2004): 944–56. https://doi.org/10.1016/j.neuropsychologia.2003.11.018.

Slimani, Maamer, David Tod, Helmi Chaabene, Bianca Miarka, and Karim Chamari. "Effects of Mental Imagery on Muscular Strength in Healthy and Patient Participants: A Systematic Review." *Journal of Sports Science & Medicine* 15, no. 3 (September 2016): 434–50. https://www.ncbi.nlm.nih.gov/pmc/articles/PMC4974856/.

University of East Anglia. "It's Official—Spending Time Outside Is Good For You." *ScienceDaily.* July 6, 2018. https://www.sciencedaily.com/ releases/2018/07/180706102842.htm.

Chapter 7

American Association of Neurological Surgeons. "Sports-Related Head Injury." https://www.aans.org/en/Patients/Neurosurgical-Conditions -and-Treatments/Sports-related-Head-Injury.

Jeff Galloway website. http://www.jeffgalloway.com/.

US Masters Swimming website. http://usms.org.

USA Track and Field. "Race Walking." http://www.usatf.org/Sports/ Race-Walking.aspx.

INDEX

Locators in **bold** indicate charts

A

Aerobic capacity
HITT training and, 31
principles of, 15
training, cardiovascular and,
19, 20
VO$_2$ max, and, 29
Aging, athletes and, 52, 56
Alcohol, athletes and, 49, 54
American Arbitration
Association, 26
Anaerobic capacity, 78, 86
Anorexia, as orthorexia, 38
Athlete's Plates, collaboration, 46,
47, 55
Avocado Chicken Salad Bites, 161
Avocado Toast, 130

B

Baked Sweet Potato Slices, 153
Bananas, 41
Bannister, Roger, 83
Behaviors, developing new, 4, 17,
94, 99
Blood sugar
HbA1C testing, 52
spikes and crashes of, 38, 43,
48, 52
Blueberries, 41
Body, listening to, 2, 5-6, 10-11
Body types, training tailored to,
61-64
Boser, Missy, 68
Brain
exercise benefits, 11, 99
nutrition, for peak functioning,
38, 40-42, 45, 47

retraining, as to mind-set,
93-94, 103
Breakfast, 125
Avocado Toast, **124,** 130
Chia Pudding, 126
Egg Cups, 128
Overnight Oats, 127
Pulled Pork Breakfast
Tacos, 129
Brown, Jeffrey, 26
Brussels Sprouts, 148
Burnette, Shanna, 27
Butternut Squash, Brussels
Sprouts, and Quinoa Salad, 151

C

Caffeine, as a training aid,
49-50, 80
Cain, Mary, 27
Carbs
as fuel for brain, 47
role of, for performance, 45, 58
Cardiovascular health, 14-15,
19-20, 64, 70
nutritional needs, 40-42
overtraining issues, 12-13
Chia Pudding, 126
Chia seeds, 40
Children, sports and, 98
Clean sport, 27, 167
Community, 1, 109
Competitive nature, 26, 56-57,
92, 110
Cool down, as part of training,
75, 77
Core strength, importance of, 79
Cortisol, stress hormone, 72

Warm-up, 75, 76–77
Warning signs, as to overtraining,
    71, 81, 165
Weight training, 66, 78–79, 80
Workout plans
    easy days, 34, 80, 84
    fartlek, **23,** 25, 30, 86
    high-intensity interval training,
        14, 30–32, 84, 170
    low-intensity, 30

Y
Yoga, 17, 34, 102

Z
Zak, Paul, 72

ACKNOWLEDGMENTS

*In many ways, this book is a celebration of the people
who challenged and empowered me to grow as
I transformed from being a committed non-runner
to a wellness fanatic and endurance coach. As I told
our stories, I was filled with gratitude for the many
ways you've each touched my life.*

*I wouldn't be a runner without Lucy Otradovec,
Amy Moddesette, and Angie Thomas, who pushed me
to run. And I wouldn't be a coach without James Kanary,
Troy Frazier, and Bert Clothier, who had the idea
for me to attend the Lydiard/Newton coaching clinic.*

*To all the Crazies past and present: Hope Hyatt,
Jen Maloney, Kaylee Griffin, Meghan Brown,
Missy Malone, Sebastien Durandeau, Shari Ashley,
and Tami Van Hofwegen. Let's run away together!*

*Thank you to my die-hard tri crew: Jill Kirkpatrick,
Kathleen Hampton, Laurie Flatt, Marcia Hurt,
Mary Lynn Thomas, Nina Tiller, Ruthie Osa,
Tina Brandt, Jane Gochis, Diane Brittain,
Julie Coleman, Ben Custer, and Coach Terry Elsmore.
May our adventures continue for decades!*

Jeana Charles, Stephanie Jurgenson,
Stephanie Leibengood, Molly Odum, Tracy Appleba,
Marcy Fitzpatrick, Bill Williams, Timm Wilson,
and Tamara Valdez. You are a significant part
of my story. You are my people.

Suzanne Proksa, Lyn Lindbergh,
and Heather Denniston. Your business mentorship
has been invaluable.

Everyone I have ever coached or who I interviewed for
the podcast or book. I have learned so much from you.
Thank you!

Rochelle Torke, my editor, this book would not
exist without you, and I so appreciate you taking
a chance on me!

And finally to my family—Abby, Sarah, Katie,
and Chris Peek. Thank you for your patience as I wrote,
avoided chores, and missed more than a few events.
This book is a dream come true and wouldn't be possible
without your love and support.

ABOUT THE AUTHOR

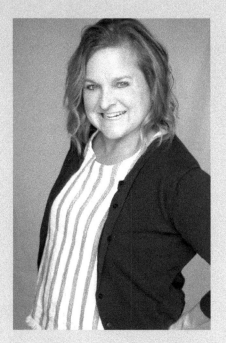

In her early 40s, Kim Peek became a runner, a triathlete, and then a coach. But she didn't always like endurance activities. At one point, she threatened to fire her trainer because their sessions involved running around the one-tenth mile track at the gym. She stuck with it because she enjoyed the camaraderie among the moms, and because she quickly dropped 50 pounds, all while realizing she was capable of achieving hard things.

Overzealous, she faced injury after injury—until she attended a coaching education program, which she participated in only because she wanted to find a way to break her own injury cycle. She came away with answers and knew she needed to teach others what she'd discovered. She has been learning from the masters and digging into research ever since.

The discipline she developed as a runner gave her the strength to face a 2015 breast cancer diagnosis with courage. She continued running through treatment and celebrated the end of chemo by running a half marathon with a group of friends a week later.

Kim has never been content with sitting back and letting life happen to her. Every obstacle, injury, and surgery motivated her to look for solutions and continue her education. On Kim's podcast,

Power Up Your Performance, she explores what it means to be a champion and interviews athletes and experts so we can all learn how to think, feel, perform, and live like champions.

Kim is a USA Track and Field Level 1 Coach, USA Triathlon Level 1 Coach, Lydiard Level II Coach, Healthy Running Coach, and RRCA Coach. She is also an ACE Certified Group Fitness Instructor, a Functional Aging Specialist, and a Breast Cancer Exercise Specialist.

Whether she's speaking, presenting a workshop, or coaching an individual athlete, Kim turns her own bumps and twists in the road of life into training plans and programs that inspire others to push their bodies and minds to achieve more than they ever imagined. You can learn more about Kim, her podcast, and her coaching programs at https://www.crushingmygoals.com.

CPSIA information can be obtained
at www.ICGtesting.com
Printed in the USA
JSHW022119130320
4670JS00003B/3